Psychoanalysis in the Technoculture Era

By now the Internet and other forms of virtual communication have been in place for at least 20 years. However, surprisingly little has been written about the use of new technologies in the psychoanalytical literature. As such, *Psychoanalysis in the Technoculture Era* is a timely exposition on the subject of both virtual and analytic space.

Bringing together the work of several psychoanalysts, the editors illustrate how new technologies have become an integral part of our everyday lives and how they have silently and subtly permeated the psychoanalytic setting. The contributors explore how new technologies have affected psychoanalytic practice and discuss the advantages and disadvantages of its use.

Psychoanalysis in the Technoculture Era unravels some of the meanings of virtual world terms, and opens this field to greater scrutiny, stimulating and promoting discussion about new technologies in psychoanalytic practice. This book will be of interest to the psychoanalytic community including psychotherapy professionals, psychoanalysts, postgraduate, graduate and undergraduate students.

Alessandra Lemma is a Fellow of the British Psychoanalytic Society, Visiting Professor in the Psychoanalysis Unit at University College London, and Visiting Professor of Psychological Therapies at Essex University. She is the Director of the Psychological Therapies Development Unit at the Tavistock and Portman NHS Trust and an Adult Psychotherapist at the Portman Clinic.

Luigi Caparrotta is a Consultant Psychiatrist in Psychotherapy and a Fellow of the British Psychoanalytical Society. He works in the NHS for Camden and Islington Foundation Trust and in private practice.

The New Library of Psychoanalysis
General Editor: Alessandra Lemma

The New Library of Psychoanalysis was launched in 1987 in association with the Institute of Psychoanalysis, London. It took over from the International Psychoanalytical Library which published many of the early translations of the works of Freud and the writings of most of the leading British and Continental psychoanalysts.

The purpose of the New Library of Psychoanalysis is to facilitate a greater and more widespread appreciation of psychoanalysis and to provide a forum for increasing mutual understanding between psychoanalysts and those working in other disciplines such as the social sciences, medicine, philosophy, history, linguistics, literature and the arts. It aims to represent different trends both in British psychoanalysis and in psychoanalysis generally. The New Library of Psychoanalysis is well placed to make available to the English-speaking world psychoanalytic writings from other European countries and to increase the interchange of ideas between British and American psychoanalysts. Through the *Teaching Series*, the New Library of Psychoanalysis now also publishes books that provide comprehensive, yet accessible, overviews of selected subject areas aimed at those studying psychoanalysis and related fields such as the social sciences, philosophy, literature and the arts.

The Institute, together with the British Psychoanalytical Society, runs a low-fee psychoanalytic clinic, organizes lectures and scientific events concerned with psychoanalysis and publishes the *International Journal of Psychoanalysis*. It runs the a training course in psychoanalysis which leads to membership of the International Psychoanalytical Association – the body which preserves internationally agreed standards of training, of professional entry, and of professional ethics and practice for psychoanalysis as initiated and developed by Sigmund Freud. Distinguished members of the Institute have included Michael Balint, Wilfred Bion, Ronald Fairbairn, Anna Freud, Ernest Jones, Melanie Klein, John Rickman and Donald Winnicott.

Previous general editors have included David Tuckett, who played a very active role in the establishment of the New Library. He was followed as general editor by Elizabeth Bott Spillius, who was in turn followed by Susan Budd and then by Dana Birksted-Breen.

ALSO IN THIS SERIES

Impasse and Interpretation Herbert Rosenfeld
Psychoanalysis and Discourse Patrick Mahony
The Suppressed Madness of Sane Men Marion Milner
The Riddle of Freud Estelle Roith
Thinking, Feeling, and Being Ignacio Matte Blanco
The Theatre of the Dream Salomon Resnik
Melanie Klein Today: Volume 1, Mainly Theory Edited by Elizabeth Bott Spillius
Melanie Klein Today: Volume 2, Mainly Practice Edited by Elizabeth Bott Spillius
Psychic Equilibrium and Psychic Change: Selected Papers of Betty Joseph Edited by Michael Feldman and Elizabeth Bott Spillius
About Children and Children-No-Longer: Collected Papers 1942–80 Paula Heimann. Edited by Margret Tonnesmann
The Freud–Klein Controversies 1941–45 Edited by Pearl King and Riccardo Steiner
Dream, Phantasy and Art Hanna Segal
Psychic Experience and Problems of Technique Harold Stewart
Clinical Lectures on Klein & Bion Edited by Robin Anderson
From Fetus to Child Alessandra Piontelli
A Psychoanalytic Theory of Infantile Experience: Conceptual and Clinical Reflections E Gaddini. Edited by Adam Limentani
The Dream Discourse Today Edited and introduced by Sara Flanders
The Gender Conundrum: Contemporary Psychoanalytic Perspectives on Feminitity and Masculinity Edited and introduced by Dana Breen
Psychic Retreats John Steiner
The Taming of Solitude: Separation Anxiety in Psychoanalysis Jean-Michel Quinodoz
Unconscious Logic: An Introduction to Matte-Blanco's Bi-logic and its Uses Eric Rayner
Understanding Mental Objects Meir Perlow
Life, Sex and Death: Selected Writings of William Gillespie Edited and introduced by Michael Sinason
What Do Psychoanalysts Want?: The Problem of Aims in Psychoanalytic Therapy Joseph Sandler and Anna Ursula Dreher
Michael Balint: Object Relations, Pure and Applied Harold Stewart
Hope: A Shield in the Economy of Borderline States Anna Potamianou

Psychoanalysis, Literature & War: Papers 1972–1995 Hanna Segal
Emotional Vertigo: Between Anxiety and Pleasure Danielle Quinodoz
Early Freud and Late Freud Ilse Grubrich-Simitis
A History of Child Psychoanalysis Claudine and Pierre Geissmann
Belief and Imagination: Explorations in Psychoanalysis Ronald Britton
A Mind of One's Own: A Psychoanalytic View of Self and Object Robert A Caper
Psychoanalytic Understanding of Violence and Suicide Edited by Rosine Jozef Perelberg
On Bearing Unbearable States of Mind Ruth Riesenberg-Malcolm
Psychoanalysis on the Move: The Work of Joseph Sandler Edited by Peter Fonagy, Arnold M. Cooper and Robert S. Wallerstein
The Dead Mother: The Work of André Green Edited by Gregorio Kohon
The Fabric of Affect in the Psychoanalytic Discourse André Green
The Bi-Personal Field: Experiences of Child Analysis Antonino Ferro
The Dove that Returns, the Dove that Vanishes: Paradox and Creativity in Psychoanalysis Michael Parsons
Ordinary People, Extra-ordinary Protections: A Post Kleinian Approach to the Treatment of Primitive Mental States Judith Mitrani
The Violence of Interpretation: From Pictogram to Statement Piera Aulagnier
The Importance of Fathers: A Psychoanalytic Re-Evaluation Judith Trowell and Alicia Etchegoyen
Dreams That Turn Over a Page: Paradoxical Dreams in Psychoanalysis Jean-Michel Quinodoz
The Couch and the Silver Screen: Psychoanalytic Reflections on European Cinema Andrea Sabbadini
In Pursuit of Psychic Change: The Betty Joseph Workshop Edited by Edith Hargreaves and Arturo Varchevker
The Quiet Revolution in American Psychoanalysis: Selected Papers of Arnold M. Cooper Arnold M. Cooper, Edited and Introduced by Elizabeth L. Auchincloss
Seeds of Illness and Seeds of Recovery: The Genesis of Suffering and the Role of Psychoanalysis Antonino Ferro
The Work of Psychic Figurability: Mental States Without Representation César Botella and Sára Botella
Key Ideas for a Contemporary Psychoanalysis: Misrecognition and Recognition of the Unconscious André Green
The Telescoping of Generations: Listening to the Narcissistic Links Between Generations Haydée Faimberg
Glacial Times: A Journey through the World of Madness Salomon Resnik
This Art of Psychoanalysis: Dreaming Undreamt Dreams and Interrupted Cries Thomas H. Ogden
Psychoanalysis and Religion in the 21st Century: Competitors or Collaborators? David M. Black
Recovery of the Lost Good Object Eric Brenman

The Many Voices of Psychoanalysis Roger Kennedy
Feeling the Words: Neuropsychoanalytic Understanding of Memory and the Unconscious Mauro Mancia
Constructions and the Analytic Field: History, Scenes and Destiny Domenico Chianese
Projected Shadows: Psychoanalytic Reflections on the Representation of Loss in European Cinema Edited by Andrea Sabbadini
Encounters with Melanie Klein: Selected Papers of Elizabeth Spillius Elizabeth Spillius
Yesterday, Today and Tomorrow Hanna Segal
Psychoanalysis Comparable and Incomparable: The Evolution of a Method to Describe and Compare Psychoanalytic Approaches David Tuckett, Roberto Basile, Dana Birksted-Breen, Tomas Böhm, Paul Denis, Antonino Ferro, Helmut Hinz, Arne Jemstedt, Paola Mariotti and Johan Schubert
Time, Space and Phantasy Rosine Jozef Perelberg
Rediscovering Psychoanalysis: Thinking and Dreaming, Learning and Forgetting Thomas H. Ogden
Mind Works: Techniques and Creativity in Psychoanalysis Antonino Ferro
Doubt Conviction and the Analytic Process: Selected Papers of Michael Feldman Michael Feldman
Melanie Klein in Berlin: Her First Psychoanalyses of Children Claudia Frank
The Psychotic Wavelength: A Psychoanalytic Perspective for Psychiatry Richard Lucas
Betweenity: A Discussion of the Concept of Borderline Judy Gammelgaard
The Intimate Room: Theory and Technique of the Analytic Field Giuseppe Civitarese
Bion Today Edited by Chris Mawson
Secret Passages: The Theory and Technique of Interpsychic Relations Stefano Bolognini
Intersubjective Processes and the Unconscious: An Integration of Freudian, Kleinian and Bionian Perspectives Lawrence J. Brown
Seeing and Being Seen: Emerging from a Psychic Retreat John Steiner
Avoiding Emotions, Living Emotions Antonio Ferro
Projective Identification: The Fate of a Concept Edited by Elizabeth Spillius and Edna O'Shaughnessy
Creative Readings: Essays on Seminal Analytic Works Thomas Ogden
The Maternal Lineage Edited by Paola Mariotti
Donald Winnicott Today Edited by Jan Abram
Symbiosis and Ambiguity: A Psychoanalytic Study Edited by John Churcher, José Bleger and Leopoldo Bleger
Psychotic Temptation Liliane Abensour
Supervision in Psychoanalysis: The Sao Paulo Seminars Antonino Ferro
Transference and Countertransference Today Robert Oelsner

TITLES IN THE NEW LIBRARY OF PSYCHOANALYSIS TEACHING SERIES

Reading Freud: A Chronological Exploration of Freud's Writings Jean-Michel Quinodoz
Listening to Hanna Segal: Her Contribution to Psychoanalysis Jean-Michel Quinodoz
Reading French Psychoanalysis Edited by Dana Birksted-Breen, Sara Flanders and Alain Gibeault
Reading Winnicott Lesley Caldwell and Angela Joyce
Initiating Psychoanalysis: Perspectives Bernard Reith, Sven Lagerlöf, Penelope Crick, Mette Møller and Elisabeth Skale
Infant Observation Frances Salo
Reading Anna Freud Nick Midgley

TITLES IN THE NEW LIBRARY OF PSYCHOANALYSIS 'BEYOND THE COUCH' SERIES

Under the Skin: A Psychoanalytic Study of Body Modification Alessandra Lemma
Engaging with Climate Change: Psychoanalytic and Interdisciplinary Perspectives Edited by Sally Weintrobe
Research on the Couch: Single Case Studies, Subjectivity, and Psychoanalytic Knowledge R.D. Hinshelwood
Psychoanalysis in the Technoculture Era Edited by Alessandra Lemma and Luigi Caparrotta

Psychoanalysis in the Technoculture Era

Edited by
Alessandra Lemma and
Luigi Caparrotta

Routledge
Taylor & Francis Group
LONDON AND NEW YORK

First published 2014
by Routledge
27 Church Road, Hove, East Sussex BN3 2FA

Simultaneously published in the USA and Canada
by Routledge
711 Third Avenue, New York, NY 10017

Routledge is an imprint of the Taylor & Francis Group, an informa business

British Library Cataloguing in Publication Data
A catalogue record for this book is available from the British Library

Library of Congress Cataloging in Publication Data
Psychoanalysis in the technoculture era / edited by Alessandra Lemma and Luigi Caparrotta.
pages cm
Includes bibliographical references.
1. Psychoanalysis—Information technology. 2. Medical innovations.
3. Mental illness—Treatment. I. Lemma, Alessandra. II. Caparrotta, Luigi.
RC504.P753 2013
616.89'1700285—dc23 2013000557

ISBN: 978-0-415-65671-9 (hbk)
ISBN: 978-0-415-65672-6 (pbk)
ISBN: 978-0-203-75833-5 (ebk)

Typeset in Garamond
by Cenveo Publisher Services

MIX
Paper from responsible sources
FSC
www.fsc.org
FSC® C013056

Printed and bound in Great Britain by
TJ International Ltd, Padstow, Cornwall

To Martin, Thomas and Matteo

Contents

Contributors

Vincenzo Bonaminio, PhD is a training and supervising analyst and a full member of the Italian Psychoanalytic Society. He works in private practice with adults and children in Rome. He is Adjunct Professor at Sapienza, University of Rome, and Visiting Professor at the Psychoanalysis Unit, University College London. He is Director of Winnicott Centro, Rome and of the *iW* – Istituto Winnicott – a five-year training programme in Child, Adolescent, and Couple Psychoanalytic Psychotherapy associated with the Department of Child and Adolescent Psychiatry, Sapienza, University of Rome. He has been Vice-President of the European Psychoanalytic Federation (EPF). He has published extensively.

Luigi Caparrotta, MD, MPhil is a consultant psychiatrist in Psychotherapy and a Fellow of the British Psychoanalytical Society. He works in the NHS for Camden and Islington Foundation Trust and in private practice. He has published a number of papers on clinical issues including the shame effect and psychotherapy assessment. He is a founding member of the British–Italian Psychoanalytical Dialogue.

Glen Gabbard, MD, is Clinical Professor of Psychiatry at Baylor College of Medicine in Houston; Professor of Psychiatry at State University of New York – Upstate Medical University in Syracuse, New York; and Training and Supervising Analyst, Center for Psychoanalytic Studies in Houston. He was Joint Editor-in-Chief of the International Journal of Psychoanalysis from 2001–2007, the first non-British Editor. He is the author or editor of 27 books, including *Textbook of Psychoanalysis*, *Love and Hate in the Analytic Setting*, and *Boundaries and Boundary Violations in Psychoanalysis*. He has received numerous awards, including the Mary Sigourney Award in 2000 for outstanding contributions to psychoanalysis.

Florence Guignard is a member of the Société Psychanalytique de Paris and full member of the International Psychoanalytical Society. She is currently the Chair of the IPA COCAP (Committee on Child and Adolescent Psychoanalysis) of which she has been a member since its foundation.

In 1997 she was elected directly by the IPA as a Child Analyst. Together with Annie Anzieu, she created the Association pour la Psychanalyse de l'Enfant (APE) in 1983, and in 1993 a European structure, the Société pour la Psychanalyse de l'Enfant et de l'Adolescent (SEPEA). She is currently the President of that society, which has articulate by-laws and a linkage with the IPA through the identity of its members. She was the head and remains a member of the Editorial Board of *L'Année Psychanalytique Internationale*, a publication in French of the International Journal of Psychoanalysis. She has published more than 250 papers and three books.

Alessandra Lemma is a consultant clinical psychologist and psychoanalyst. She is a Fellow of the British Psychoanalytic Society, the Director of the Psychological Therapies Development Unit at the Tavistock and Portman NHS Foundation Trust and Consultant Adult Psychotherapist at the Portman Clinic. She is also the Clinical Director of the Psychological Interventions Research Centre at University College London. She is the General Editor of the New Library of Psychoanalysis Book Series and Regional Editor (London) of the International Journal of Psychoanalysis. She is Honorary Professor of Psychological Therapies, Essex University and Visiting Professor, Psychoanalysis Unit, University College London.

Andrea Sabbadini, C. Psychol. is a Fellow of the British Psychoanalytical Society, its former Honorary Secretary and its current Director of Publications. He works in private practice in London, is a senior lecturer at UCL, a trustee of the Freud Museum, a member of the IPA Committee on Psychoanalysis and Culture, the Director of the European Psychoanalytic Film Festival and the Chairman of a programme of films and discussions at the ICA.
He is the founding editor of *Psychoanalysis and History* and the Film Section editor of *The International Journal of Psychoanalysis*. He has published in the major psychoanalytic journals, and has edited *Il tempo in psicoanalisi* (1979), *Even Paranoids Have Enemies* (1998), *The Couch and the Silver Screen* (2003), *Projected Shadows* (2007) and *Psychoanalytic Visions of Cinema* (2007).

Jill Savege Scharff, MD, MRCPsych is Supervising Analyst and founding Chair at the International Institute for Psychoanalytic Training at the International Psychotherapy Institute in Chevy Chase, Maryland, USA; Teaching Analyst at the Washington Center for Psychoanalysis, and Clinical Professor of Psychiatry at Georgetown University, Washington DC. She is a psychoanalyst in private practice with adults, children, couples and families. She has published extensively, including *Projective and Introjective Identification and the Use of the Therapist's Self* (1992), *The Interpersonal Unconscious* (2011), *Tuning the Therapeutic Instrument: Affective Learning of Psychotherapy* (2000), *Object Relations Individual Therapy* (1998), *Object*

Relations Therapy of Physical and Sexual Trauma (1996) and *The Primer of Object Relations: Second Edition* (2005).

Heather Wood is a Clinical Psychologist and Psychoanalytic Psychotherapist, and a member of the British Association of Psychotherapists. She works as Consultant Adult Psychotherapist at the Portman Clinic, Tavistock and Portman NHS Foundation Trust, a state-funded outpatient forensic psychotherapy clinic; she also works in private practice. She specialises in work with people who compulsively use legal and illegal Internet pornography and has published on Internet pornography, paedophilia and related topics.

Foreword

"*Plus ça change, plus c'est la même chose*" (Jean-Baptiste Alphonse Karr, January 1849 issue of his journal *Les Guêpes*). Or perhaps it is not true that nothing changes with change. Perhaps there are technological and social changes that cause such dramatic shifts in the way we think that there can be no return to the 'old ways'. Has the technological revolution of information technology brought about an irreversible shift in our psychological world? Has the explosion of information technology over the past 25 years changed the human condition beyond comparability with previous epochs? If so, how do these changes interface with what is unchangeable about the human condition? This is what Lemma and Caparrotta's book is trying to fathom in mapping the psychological changes implied by the introduction of information technology. The full appreciation of the profound nature of the social and psychic changes they document requires contextualizing their explorations in the biological foundations of the human culture turned upside down by the information revolution.

While biology is not destiny for the human primate, progress in behavioral and molecular genetics over the quarter-century of the information revolution has underscored for all of us that our biology places massive constraints upon what any one of us can hope to achieve or is likely to become. There is something somewhat paradoxical about a psychoanalytic exploration of this revolution of human experience. The Internet, computers, and smartphones push us to the furthest edge of progress and modernity. The glut of information on the Internet is already beyond imagination: 550 billion web-connected documents with 100,000 times as many intersections as there are on roads in the United States. Laptops now have the power of the supercomputers of two decades ago but will themselves soon be replaced by smartphones, which provide an interface with most aspects of life (such as working, eating, and religion). From the stance of the psychoanalyst this perplexing progress is observed against a background of what is considered most invariable and unchangeable in human nature – the timeless unconscious, repressed parts of the mind, the product of what is discussed as inborn, genetically coded, species-specific or instinctual. This is unchanging – or is it?

In György Gergely's informal analysis of biological models of mental health relying on the notion of instinct, three approaches are identified (Gergely & Jacob, 2012). The earliest psychoanalytic approach emphasized sexual and aggressive instincts as the behavioral system implicated in most emotional and behavioral abnormalities (Freud, 1905, 1915). Following the partial discrediting of the psychosexual model of mental health (e.g., Peterfreund, 1971), the instinct for attachment, giving rise to a drive for relating, started to occupy the foreground of psychodynamic thinking. This was perhaps initiated by the work of John Bowlby (1960), but came to be integrated with the instincts of sexuality and aggression in the writings of object relations theorists (Fairbairn, 1952; Kernberg, 1976). More recently, some psychoanalytic writers alighted on what may be considered an instinct for communication and interpersonal understanding (Fonagy, 2003). The instinct for orienting towards others to learn about the self has been added as a further biological facet of emotional and behavioral growth (Tronick, 2007).

The need for the third instinctual model arises because of limitations inherent to the first two. A model of development and disturbance based on the instincts of sex and aggression failed ultimately because it could not bear the weight of complexity that was placed upon it. While it is undoubtedly true that no human being is free of conflict in these domains, it is hard not to see as reductionistic any attempt to provide accounts of the almost infinite variety of emotional and behavioral disturbance we, as a species, are capable of manifesting solely in terms of a failure to reconcile these biological drives with societal demands.

Similarly, attachment theory has only partially fulfilled its promise to provide a generic account of abnormal behavior and emotion. Relationship problems are inevitably entailed in all psychological disturbances. Trying to reduce current difficulties to disruptions of early attachment is clearly helpful as a heuristic to elaborate such problems. It has proved to be quite disappointing in causal accounts, as early attachment fails to account for much variance in the emergence of later emotional difficulties (Fearon, Bakermans-Kranenburg, Van IJzendoorn, Lapsley, & Roisman, 2010). Separation, for example, had promise as a key indicator of the frustration of the drive for attachment leading to later disturbance, but this hope has not been borne out by longitudinal studies, where in a great number of instances early adversity did not lead to later disturbance (Ollendick, Costa, & Benoit, 2010).

This brings us to the instinct for communication, which is perhaps the only one of this triad that is genuinely specific to our species (Sperber & Wilson, 2012; Tomasello, 2005). Core to our humanity is the transmission of knowledge and beliefs from one generation to the next. What is (sometimes perhaps somewhat confusingly) referred to as 'culture' is made up of essential pieces of information about the use of objects we as a species have created and refined. We have tools for producing food, pleasure, and providing protection. We also have belief systems that connect us to the physical environment that we find ourselves in. Culture is the collective noun used to describe information that each human newborn has to acquire if they are to take a productive role in their specific social environment. To preserve their genes (Hamilton, 1964) and their position in relation to their environment, our ancestors needed to transmit their knowledge, and evolved a communication system that has as its primary function the instruction of young humans in the nature of the world.

A human-specific, cue-driven social–cognitive adaptation of mutual design has evolved, dedicated to ensuring the efficient transfer of relevant cultural knowledge (Csibra & Gergely, 2009, 2011; Gergely, Kiraly, & Egyed, 2007). Humans are predisposed to 'teach' and 'learn' new and relevant cultural information from each other. The pedagogic stance is the attitude adopted by an individual wishing to teach a young human about some aspect of reality. Some information we are able to accept because of its content. We grasp the deductive relations of the new information to the contents of other beliefs. Alternatively, we appraise its usefulness and veracity by establishing inductive relations to the evidence, in accordance with the principles of theoretical rationality. However, mostly there is little evidence available, and new information may not link well with the network of prior beliefs. Thus, the transmission of information occurs largely by an alternative path, and veracity is established by authority: its source is known, remembered, and judged to be reliable (or trustworthy). We may say that information that is taken to be shared common knowledge among members of one's community is largely 'deferentially' transmitted (Recanati, 1997). The acceptance of authority is initiated by a special set of cues with which the adult signals that the next piece of information is relevant to the addressee generally rather than specifically to the emergent situation.

Such cues, labeled *ostensive cues* in the Theory of Natural Pedagogy (Csibra & Gergely, 2006), are instinctual – biologically prepared. They are understood from infancy and include addressing the individual directly with eye contact, repeating their name, using special intonation, and responding appropriately and sensitively to their actions and expressions, with the teacher titrating his or her behavior to moment-to-moment changes in the addressee's state. From early infancy these cues trigger a different quality of attention in the addressee, who listens and encodes the content of communication as generically relevant (i.e., potentially part of what must be learnt about culture). Language *per se* may be the product of this imperative to teach. The need for culture arises only when tools become the primary means of survival (Gergely & Jacob, in press). But tools are opaque in their function, and their use must be acquired through demonstration and description. It is possible – some have argued – that the gestures initially used for demonstration of states of mind in relation to the use of tools gradually become gestures of sound, where oral mimicry took the place of physical mimicry (Fónagy, 2000; Fónagy & Fonagy, 1995). Ultimately, this then gives rise to another form of communication, where sounds are stripped of their iconic significance and become symbols rather than signals. The instinct for communication, of course, underpins this evolutionary path.

Acquiring the culture through language, as well as prelinguistic modes of learning, is thus biologically primed. Evolution has created an *epistemic superhighway*, which facilitates the transmission of knowledge. While the new technologies may on the surface interact to some degree with the first two forms of evolutionary-protected instinctual functions, it is in this third territory where this impact is most profound. No doubt Internet sex and violent video games give alternative expressions to sex and aggression, the biological drives that we share with most other living organisms. Tumblr, Twitter, YouTube, and dozens of other social networking media are likely to build new mechanisms around the creation of relationships and their maintenance across space and time (witness the popularity of Facebook or Friends Reunited). Once more, however, attachment as a process is unaffected by these new modalities for its expression, and ultimately the programs for maintaining relationships electronically represent superstructural modifications of the biological process. The underlying instinctual functions are unaffected; new expressions may be found, and perhaps in the cases of the drives for relating these are enriched in quantity, even if perhaps not deepened.

By dramatic contrast, the third of these instincts related to the transfer of knowledge is altered in its essence, not just in its expression or its manifestations. The evolutionarily carefully protected mechanism for transmitting information by human communication is modified by information technology. Communication depends on *trust*. Evolution protects us from being misled by malicious agents who have interests other than ours in mind and may transmit false information. *Deferentially transmitted* information is protected by the use of ostensive cues – the interaction whereby the teacher establishes credibility with the addressee or student by responding sensitively, with careful matching of her or his actions to those of the student. Media, film, and television represented a threat to this process of cultural transmission, but none of these is able to replicate the key that opens the human mind to influence, the presence of someone who has our mind in mind, someone responding to us contingently, whose interest in us serves as a trigger for our interest in what they have to say.

Information technology, however, can simulate the *pedagogic stance*. The messaging of modern information technology is complicated from an evolutionary psychology standpoint because it *can* mold itself around the addressee. We are open to receive, believe, and retransmit messages that might normally leave us unaffected because we feel they are addressed directly at us by 'someone' with immediate concern for our wellbeing. '*Big Data*' can monitor our interests, deliver advertisements specific to our taste and previous responses, create novels that unfold at the rate of our reading speed, identify ideas and thoughts – perhaps even feelings – that we are likely to orient towards.

If this sounds like Big Brother, it is exactly that – even if 25 years later than anticipated.

Potentially, the sensitivity of the Internet 'to our needs' is far greater than the most caring and concerned adult could possibly be. The processing power of supercomputers permits *all* human beings to be accurately recognized and mirrored by Bayesian algorithms. This, perhaps more than anything else, demands that we carefully study the relationship of person and machine from the point of view of subjective experience. This is the road that Lemma and Caparrotta have set out on, and it behoves us to accompany them on this journey – perhaps the most important intellectual journey to be undertaken this decade. We should think about human subjectivity in the face of information technology in the context of pedagogy and its evolutionary role in cultural transmission. We are, as a species, biologically vulnerable to what the Internet has to offer: individual attention.

This is why Lemma and Caparrotta's book is vital. It is perhaps a first attempt at exploring, with knowledge of the unconscious as well as the conscious layers of subjectivity, the association between human instincts and information technology. It may be one of the first, but many more such inquiries should be undertaken so we can formulate our questions about regulation and control of the Internet in an informed and appropriate manner. There is an obvious opportunity to enhance what is most distinctively human – not sex, aggression, or relatedness, but communication and information transmission – via the Internet. The risks to us, however, are perhaps greater in this domain than in the other biological preoccupations. Persuasive messaging about suicide, self-harm, extreme dieting, or radical faiths already surrounds us with available, easily digested information presented via a medium that we are primed to internalize and accept as our own. And surely this is just the beginning. Let us hope it is not also a precipitous end. We evidently have to be watchful, but we also know that paranoia cannot be the answer.

Professor Peter Fonagy, PhD, DipPsy, FBPSA, FBA
Director, UCLPartners Mental Health and
Wellbeing Programme
Freud Memorial Professor of Psychoanalysis
Head of the Research Department of Clinical,
Educational and Health Psychology
University College London
1–19 Torrington Place
London WC1E 7HB

References

Bowlby, J. (1960). Grief and mourning in infancy and early childhood. *Psychoanalytic Study of the Child, 15*, 3–39.

Csibra, G., & Gergely, G. (2006). Social learning and social cognition: The case for pedagogy. In M. H. Johnson & Y. M. Munakata (Eds.), *Processes of change in brain and cognitive development. Attention and Performance* (Vol. XXI, pp. 249–274). Oxford: Oxford University Press.

Csibra, G., & Gergely, G. (2009). Natural pedagogy. *Trends in Cognitive Sciences, 13*, 148–153.

Csibra, G., & Gergely, G. (2011). Natural pedagogy as evolutionary adaptation. *Philosophical Transactions of the Royal Society B: Biological Sciences, 366*, 1149–1157.

Fairbairn, W. R. D. (1952). *An object-relations theory of the personality*. New York, NY: Basic Books.

Fearon, R. M. P., Bakermans-Kranenburg, M. J., Van IJzendoorn, M. H., Lapsley, A., & Roisman, M. (2010). The significance of insecure attachment and disorganization in the development of children's externalizing behavior: A meta-analytic study. *Child Development, 81*, 435–456.

Fónagy, I. (2000). *Languages within language: An evolutive approach*. Amsterdam: John Benjamins.

Fónagy, I., & Fonagy, P. (1995). Communication with pretend actions in language, literature and psychoanalysis. *Psychoanalysis and Contemporary Thought, 18*, 363–418.

Fonagy, P. (2003). Genetics, developmental psychopathology and psychoanalytic theory: The case for ending our (not so) splendid isolation. *Psychoanalytic Inquiry, 23*, 218–247.

Freud, S. (1905). Three essays on the theory of sexuality. In J. Strachey (Ed.), *The standard edition of the complete psychological works of Sigmund Freud* (Vol. 7, pp. 123–230). London: Hogarth Press.

Freud, S. (1915). Instincts and their vicissitudes. In J. Strachey (Ed.), *The standard edition of the complete psychological works of Sigmund Freud* (Vol. 14, pp. 109–140). London: Hogarth Press.

Gergely, G., & Jacob, P. (2012). Reasoning about instrumental and communicative agency in human infancy. In F. Xu & T. Kushnir (Eds.), *Advances in child development and behavior, Vol. 43: Rational constructivism in cognitive development* (pp. 59–94). London: Academic Press.

Gergely, G., Kiraly, I., & Egyed, K. (2007). On pedagogy. *Developmental Science, 10*, 139–146.

Hamilton, W. D. (1964). The genetic evolution of social behaviour. *Journal of Theoretical Biology, 7*, 1–52.

Kernberg, O. F. (1976). *Object relations theory and clinical psychoanalysis*. New York, NY: Jason Aronson.

Ollendick, T. H., Costa, N. M., & Benoit, K. E. (2010). Interpersonal processes and the anxiety disorders of childhood. In J. G. Beck (Ed.), *Interpersonal processes in the anxiety disorders: Implications for understanding psychopathology and treatment* (pp. 71–95). Washington, DC: American Psychological Association.

Peterfreund, E. (1971). *Information, systems and psychoanalysis (Psychological Issues Monograph)*. New York, NY: International Universities Press.

Recanati, F. (1997). Can we believe what we do not understand? *Mind and Language, 12*, 84–100.

Sperber, D., & Wilson, D. B. (2012). *Relevance and meaning*. Cambridge, UK: Cambridge University Press.

Tomasello, M. (2005). *Constructing a language: A usage-based theory of language acquisition*. Cambridge, MA: Harvard University Press.

Tronick, E. (2007). *The neurobehavioral and social-emotional development of infants and children*. New York, NY: W.W. Norton & Company.

Acknowledgements

This book was conceived following the 6th British–Italian Dialogue in London in 2011, whose theme was Dream Space and Virtual Space in the Analytic Situation. We therefore wish to acknowledge the contributions of the various speakers who inspired us to explore and take forward the issue of techno-culture within the psychoanalytic domain. We also wish to thank the contributors of this book, who made it possible to initiate a lively and interesting discussion on this subject, which is still controversial, poorly researched and not yet fully understood.

Many thanks to the *Journal of the American Psychoanalytic Association*, the *International Journal of Psychoanalysis* and *Psychoanalytic Quarterly* for permission to reprint articles by Alessandra Lemma, Jill Scharff and Glen Gabbard respectively.

Introduction

Luigi Caparrotta and Alessandra Lemma

"*New IPhone application lets user confess while on the go*" (Reuters, 10th February, 2011). Not long after this announcement, the Vatican issued a statement saying that the presence of a penitent and priest "cannot be substituted by any IT application … and … although God is everywhere … it is probably not in your mobile phone". While the news immediately excited some Catholics in the United States, it soon produced dissent and outrage in other Catholic countries. If we keep in mind the allergic reaction shared by many psychoanalytically trained practitioners, for example, when online therapeutic interventions are discussed, it could be said that a significant proportion of therapists and analysts might be inclined to agree with the sentiment behind the Vatican's riposte. Within our analytic communities, we can all too easily find colleagues who relate to technological developments and their use in the analytic setting (e.g. the use of texts or email, Skype analysis, online therapeutic interventions) with the same guardedness, if not outrage, of the Catholics faced with the development of the new Iphone app.

Considering that the Internet and other forms of virtual communication have been in place for at least 20 years or so, surprisingly little has been written about the use of new technologies in the psychoanalytical literature. Yet, even within clinical psychoanalysis, several psychoanalysts over the years have been using various forms of communication for supervision or treatment, including correspondence (Hofling, 1979), tape-recorders (Lindon et al., 1972), telephone, (Rosenbaum, 1977; Lindon, 1988; Leffert, 2003) and more recently emails, videos and Skype.[1] A recent preliminary survey of psychoanalysts' practice (N= 62) carried out by the British Psychoanalytic Society revealed that 31 per cent of respondents had conducted telephone/Skype analysis (Fornari-Spoto, 2011). An interesting, albeit controversial, comment to this survey was made by Symington (2011), suggesting that for those analysts "whose foundation rests upon the instincts" this gives rise to ossification and restricted communication, whereby the analytic process is seen to require the physical presence of analyst and patient in the consulting room. Those analysts "whose foundation rests on communication" tend to remain open to its various forms, including Skype or telephone. Clearly not all patients can be treated in these modified forms of analysis or psychotherapy. However, what Symington appears to be suggesting is that it may not only be that some patients are unsuitable, but also that some analysts cannot make good use of these new media.

Those analysts who do use new technologies to communicate with and treat patients, for example via texts and emails, or those bold enough to have braved Skype analysis, are nevertheless careful not to advertise the fact too widely, with a few notable exceptions (Ermann, 2004; Carlino, 2010; Lingiardi, 2008; Dini, 2009; Bonaminio, 2010; Fiorentini, 2011; Kilborne, 2011). Consequently, the literature in this area is very scarce indeed, relative to the place new technologies command in our personal and professional lives.

There is a degree of reticence to write about these changing practices. For example, we struggled at first to find a psychoanalyst willing to write a chapter on Skype analysis for this book even though we all probably know of colleagues who are receiving such analysis and/or colleagues who are delivering it. The reasons given all sounded plausible enough (e.g. 'I have not worked in this way long enough to know what I really think about it'), but the difficulty we encountered in this respect is of note. Jill Scharff, however, has contributed a helpful chapter on this subject for this edition, sharing her experience of doing telephone/Skype analysis, underlining that in many respects there is little difference between so-called teleanalysis and traditional analysis in the actual work done during the session. The dilemmas facing the analyst when working in this way are well captured by Andrea Sabbadini (this edition) drawing attention to how changing the setting to accommodate new technologies raises the thorny question of what constitutes "true" analysis, arguing that "psychoanalysis as such" can be allowed a modicum of flexibility so long as we are able to maintain the analytic stance.

Nothwithstanding Scharff's and Sabbadini's contributions, the gap between actual practice and publications on this matter may reflect a number of processes. The disparity between the older and younger (psychoanalytical) generations has inescapably created a gap between those who grew up in the world of cyberspace and those who did not. However, it must be acknowledged that this gap is gradually narrowing while some of the 'elders', grappling with the world of cyberspace, have been making room for the new psychoanalytic 'net' generation. Those analysts who are computer/Internet illiterate or semi-literate may nevertheless experience a degree of shame. Shame can undermine curiosity about these new developments, which may then be ignored, or worse still, they may be admonished as corrupting the analytic setting.

There may also be an unconscious or preconscious need to be in control, rigidity and contrariness on the part of the analyst, or even sheer contempt may be present in those analysts who dislike interference with the way they trained. Some may become concerned with any 'transference contamination' or what they regard as threats to the analytic relationship. Some may even object to the idea of being at the mercy of such 'external forces'.

In this book we suggest that communication technologies ought to be of great interest to contemporary psychoanalytic practitioners. The very existence of communication networks that facilitate and regulate intimacy, with varying degrees of connection and disconnection, strikes at the heart of what we painstakingly try to understand with our patients in our daily practices: how to manage being-with-self-and-others. In so far as these technologies have the *potential* to perform such important psychic functions, it is incumbent on us to distinguish between the "properties of tools" and "what people do with them" (Chartier, 1997: 11). It is the latter that concerns us primarily in this book. We need to understand more about how these new technologies interact with the prerogatives of an individual's internal world (see Bonaminio; Lemma; Wood, this edition), how they may alter psychic structure itself in fundamental ways (see Guignard, this edition) and the implications of this for the individual's functioning and also for how a society operates. As the sociologist Kevin Robins suggests, we need to understand how new technologies may be "mobilised to secure a detached kind of engagement – a remote-control relationship – with the world" (2001: 533). While he agrees that technological revolutions create new possibilities, the way the experience of distance and proximity can now be manipulated through various media may also be misused, a point we shall return to throughout this book. At a social level we need to be mindful of the way technologies can play into the "social production of indifference" (Herzfeld, 1992) rooted in processes of denial and disavowal that can be more or less consciously supported through the distancing mechanisms that virtual communication makes possible like never before.

New technological spaces

New technologies have changed fundamental aspects of how we learn and work in many disciplines and domains of life. Electronic learning (E-learning),[2] for example, has become a standard interactive tool in many teaching institutions. More recently telehealthcare-based interventions,[3] including virtual hospitals, are also rapidly increasing and clearly raising concerns about the alteration, if not the total absence, of the much valued doctor–patient relationship (McLean et al., 2011).

Because the individuals we see in our daily practices may be 'misusing' new technologies to manage, for example, their relationship to reality, it is all too easy to adopt a dystopic view of these developments. More generally, when faced with the so-called 'new', it is not uncommon to adopt a sceptical position. However the aura of futurology that often accompanies discussions of virtual reality runs counter to the fact that these "emblems of modernity" (Fischer, 2007) turn out not be so 'new' after all. Instead of being a quantum leap in communication one could argue that the Internet, for example, is another form of communication that merely collates and rebrands historical modes of association in order to enhance and distribute knowledge and information. We can do all the things we have always done, for example convene, converse, plan and so on, without ever having to leave our room. Koch and Lockwood (2010) have cogently pointed this out, adding that the Internet does not transcend the radical and emancipating impact of the printing press.

Any historical perspective soon exposes how these so-called 'new' technologies are part of an ongoing process of development in communications media, as was the case with the development of print and the telephone system in their respective inceptions, which dramatically altered community life and social relations. As Bingham (1996) suggests, in Victorian and Edwardian societies, the advent of the telephone challenged the established patterns of privacy and hierarchy because it facilitated immediate communication. It is indeed this very quality of *immediacy* that distinguishes the technologies we are especially concerned with in this book. The question of how this impacts, in turn, on internalised and external object relationships – and on social relations more broadly – begs a psychoanalytic lens to be applied to these ongoing developments.

We want to make it clear from the outset, however, that our intention is neither to demonise nor to eulogise the power of media communication and information technology, or for that matter to undermine or idealise the basic psychoanalytic setting. Contributors to the book take opposing views at times, for example on whether virtual space can be conceptualised as a kind of transitional space (see chapters by Bonaminio, Guignard, and Lemma) or whether the use of technology so fundamentally shapes psychic structure and hence how we relate that we are witnessing a change in the kind of pathology we encounter in our consulting rooms. Florence Guignard takes the most polarized position in this respect, suggesting a link between the dominance of virtual modes of relating and the increase in borderline presentations especially in young people today. She argues that virtual communication fuels the expectation of immediate gratification of wishes and desires and increases the risk that the three aspects of the basic assumption group mentality (Bion, 1961) highjack thinking for oneself. More fundamentally she boldly proposes that the virtual world and other societal changes that give ascendance to the social group as opposed to the parental couple in children's early development, contribute to the erosion of a "latency period in space and time", which as psychoanalysts we have regarded as central to the development of psychic structure.

Whether there is a link between the kinds of pathology we see nowadays and technological developments or whether, say, borderline patients are more likely to be drawn to the virtual world and 'misuse' it because of their marked interpersonal difficulties is debatable. These questions are evidently ripe for discussion. We wanted to include such contrasting views because we are so early on in our understanding of these processes that we need varied, even polarised, perspectives to help us to consider from different vantage points the use made of technological developments at individual and societal levels. We are of the view, however, that precisely because we know so little about these processes, we are not in a position to generalize and we need to keep an open mind, not least because what we learn about the virtual world from the vantage point of the couch inevitably gives us a skewed perspective.

As the chapters in this book will make clear, technological 'developments' can be recruited to manage psychological problems and conflict or to manage the felt-to-be perils of intimacy in the transference relationship. But we also want to suggest that these developments are also 'developments' in the sense that they have created opportunities for extending learning and creativity that were unimaginable before the advent of the Internet. These new media also offer opportunities for increasing accessibility to psychoanalytic interventions. While this requires a sophisticated understanding of how to best create and safeguard the analytic setting, and we have much to learn in this respect, this does not mean that it is not possible to work psychoanalytically through these media (see Carlino, 2010; Lemma & Fonagy, in press; Sabbadini, this edition; Scharff, this edition).

These technologies have become an integral part of our everyday lives and of our psychoanalytic practice. We are thus keen to seize the opportunity in this book, and in this chapter in particular, to explore not only the varied uses made of new forms of technology and their psychic function in the internal world, but also to be curious about how such technological developments may help us to explore some assumptions about what we call the psychoanalytic frame.

Unravelling some of the meanings of virtual world terms

Before going any further, it is important to clarify the meaning of some of the new technological terms that will be referred to in this book. The word *cyberspace* was coined by William Gibson's novel *Neuromancer* in 1984, (Gibson, 1984) well before the Internet was launched. After conjuring up a world where reality, technology and consciousness merge into each other, he describes it as a highly complex shared form of hallucination. However, nowadays cyberspace commonly refers to any large collection of network-accessible computer-based data (Oxford dictionary, 2008). This global informal network (*Internet*) has now become the source of '*hubs* joining strong and weak links' dominating the media world. Hub, originally a central point of interest, is now used in computer parlance as indicating a place of cooperation between 'strong and weak links'.[4] It is at the heart of what is now called *social networking*, where registered members, including designated 'friends', are encouraged to upload an online personal profile in order to form a shared network of common interests. Typical examples of this networking are Facebook, MySpace and Twitter. In this way social media websites provide an intricate 'forum' or 'blog'[5] of social connections and interactions. As we are well aware, the ensuing security and privacy problems generated by these networks are considerable.

Virtual reality generally refers to the generation by computer software of an image or experience of environments that appear real to the senses, while the *virtual world* represents a world created by a program where an object (an avatar) is created and maintained to imitate a human or other being. An *avatar* is an interactive social representation of its user that can be controlled by the user and mediates interactions online. It may be likened to a "portrait" of ourselves (Meadows, 2008).

Fink firmly locates the virtual in relation to a notion of an internal world, defining the virtual as "something that exists in the mind without actual physical fact, form, or features ... virtual realities occur in inner mental space, reflecting internal environments" (1999: 22). Heim (1998) points to the origin of the word in the Latin *virtus*, meaning 'human power', thereby underlining that the virtual comes out of human creation rather than existing in the 'actual' of the physical world (Jones, 2006).

The virtual world can be conceived as a "complex reality simulation that may induce a number of emotional responses" (Riva, 2005). Within this context virtual reality can be defined as a representation of an imaginary world or environment. The individual may relate to this space in adaptive ways, but also as an unoccupied space available for the taking, fuelling omnipotent fantasies of unbridled freedom that can become intoxicating (see Lemma; Wood, this edition).

The spatial vernacular that surrounds discussions of these technologies underlines the way that cyberspace is conceptualised and experienced by many as a physical space that can be 'entered' and where people can be met and engaged with. The relationship to the machine itself is not only a psychological one, but also a physical one. When children play video games we can observe their bodies moving in line with the movements on the screen. The machine(s) can feel to the user as an extension of their bodily self. A variety of devices explicitly reinforce this subjective experience through making representations seem like an extension of the user's lived space, for example, the notion of a computer's 'desktop' can seamlessly be seen as an extension of the user's physical desk.

For a discipline like psychoanalysis – one predicated on a fundamental human tension between the lure of the 'pleasure principle' and the dampener of the "reality principle" (Freud, 1923) – the virtual is to the real what the copy is to the original: it is a reproduction that allows wishes to colonise reality. In such a definition the virtual is always 'less than' the original. The virtual omnipotently divests the so-called 'real' of its bones and flesh reality. Indeed, as Hayles aptly put it: "As we rush to explore the new vistas that cyberspace has made available for colonisation, let us also remember the fragility of a material world that cannot be replaced" (1993: 91).

The virtual, as Baudrillard declared, is the desire for "a resolution of the world ahead of time by the cloning of reality and the extermination of the real by its double" (1996: 25). Baudrillard seizes here on the omnipotent state of mind that, as clinicians, we would all too readily recognise in our work with patients who become addicted to the possibility of gratifying in real-time the internal world's wishes, not least through a denial of corporeality, a point we will return to shortly and that several of the chapters speak to (see Lemma; Wood, this edition). Indeed, "virtual technologies", writes Hillis, "encourage belief that they constitute a 'transcendence machine' within which the imaginative self might escape its privatized physical anchor and live in an iconography of pleasure" (1999: 172).

The definition of 'virtual' typically stands in opposition to the notion of 'real'. As such, thinking about the nature of virtual reality can be unhelpfully short-circuited and polarised: the virtual becomes equated with 'not authentic', a retreat away from so-called reality. As psychoanalytic practitioners, however, we are all too accustomed to the virtual nature of the real itself as it is filtered through a world of object relations – one in turn distorted by projective and introjective processes – that creates virtual others who carry emotional resonance within and inform how we experience and act in the world.

Even though virtual reality may be used to effectuate a retreat away from reality, we could equally argue for a notion of a virtuality that is not always about a 'safe copy' of, or 'alternative' to the 'real'. Jones (2006) engagingly draws on the observations of Stewart and Nicholls (2002) who describe how the English gardens of the nineteenth century were informed more by the virtual image of the painter than actual nature, and gardeners designed spaces to reflect this virtual space within the natural world:

> Just as a painter need not be constrained by 'reality' in creating the most 'natural' landscape — this can be eliminated, that can be added; this can be highlighted, that can be muted — so a gardener/architect can craft a multi-perspective view of the landscape.
>
> (Stewart & Nicholls, 2002: 94)

Jones makes the point that "the boundaries between natural/artificial, real/virtual, even nature/culture were blurred by these spaces, but they still were experienced as real" (2006: 12), and indeed they proved to be a creative inspiration for the English gardeners.

If we adopt, for example, Delueze's suggestion that "the virtual is opposed not to the real but to the actual" (1994: 208) then the virtual is fully real insofar as it is virtual. Moreover this kind of virtuality may represent a necessary step towards the realm of what is possible. In other words, it may contain the seeds for imagining oneself as different and hence for being different. Here the real may be seen as partial, flawed, while the virtual promises a resolution to come, which may then be experimented with in virtual reality before being actualised in reality.

Relating in the virtual world

Technology has slipped into our everyday lives and it is now hard to imagine life without various gadgets, which have become extensions of our bodies and hence of our selves: when we go into our offices or consulting rooms, the first thing we 'pre-consciously' do is to switch on the computer, Iphone, BlackBerry or whatever new mobile gadget we have in order to keep ourselves 'connected' to the world. Of course, the ability to 'connect' that these new technologies afford may also be rightly questioned since this so-called 'virtual' connection may erode other embodied forms of connection, as William Powers points out in *Hamlet's BlackBerry* (2010). For example, a family cannot even sit down together without one of its members taking off sooner or later in order to look at some form of a screen or another.

Technology, starting with the advent of print and then telephony, has radically transformed our ways of communicating and our spatio-temporal organisation externally as much as internally. These developments urge us to "rethink space-time" (Doel & Clarke, 2006) as they introduce new forms of relating and hence of acting in the world with others (Thomson, 1995). Through the medium of representation we can now bring remote events and people near while experiencing them at a remove (Robins, 2001). This facility may be used constructively to connect with people who are geographically distant, as well as destructively to undermine a real emotional connection with others who are physically removed and hence whose pain is not our business, as it were (see for example, the experience of war as it is filtered through our television screens).

Watching some children playing with their Nintendos, engrossed in the virtual reality it gives them access to, oblivious to all around them, can leave us in little doubt that they are encapsulated in a world all of their own. Of course, this is also true of other activities such as sports or reading. The issue here is whether any of these activities are pursued *compulsively*. For example, the fury that the withdrawal of the Nintendo can unleash in some young people could be seen as a measure of its lure in the internal world. The Nintendo, like a drug or alcohol, can substitute for less satisfactory relationships. Computers are indeed often spoken about and related to as if they were animate. The idea of a corporeal screen and processor is implicit in notions such as computer 'viruses' or 'bugs' (White, 2006).

The avatar is the perfect tool for titrating intimacy. Paradoxically, however, because of the illusion of the anonymity afforded by the mask that is the avatar, people often disclose a great deal about themselves online, far more than they would do normally. Because 'information' is more important than physical proximity in cyberspace, interactions online may then leave some vulnerable people feeling unexpectedly very exposed.[6]

The etymological roots of the term cyberspace from the Greek 'kybernan', meaning to control or steer, direct us towards an important feature of cyberspace that accounts for its lure: in that space the individual can feel in control as he manipulates reality. Whatever else cyberspace is it is also fundamentally a felt-to-be controlled space. How much easier to enter a world in which you can feel totally in control, where what you need is but one click away, where the feeding 'screen-mother' can be switched on and off at will (Lemma, this edition).

We have become so dependent on our gadgets – either as extensions of our physical and cognitive boundaries or as psychic retreats (Steiner, 1993) when they acquire a more rigid and/or compulsive function in the internal world – that it is hardly surprising that we experience a terrible sense of loss and deprivation when they get lost or they 'crash' (Lingiardi, 2008). Such 'failures' provide a different narrative to the one about the 'control' afforded by the technology. The machine's failure exposes the helplessness concealed behind the fantasy of control. However, the notion that new technologies allow for the possibility of an escape from normative identities, whereby at the click of a prostheses (e.g. the mouse) people can switch sex or class, cannot be considered, as Cohen (2001) notes, in isolation from its counterpart, namely that the individual is regulated by the very technologies that simulate freedom from the constraints of reality, and in particular, of the given body.

For some individuals the 'dependency' on technology may acquire a more compelling quality to such an extent that, without access to the technology and the access to virtual reality that it affords, the sense of self fragments. We cannot simply comment from the perspective of the consulting room, as it were, to understand these kinds of internal processes because they are, inevitably, in a dynamic interaction or tension with external socio-cultural processes, which reinforce – even normalise – psychic defensive strategies. The relentless emphasis on transformation and change dominant now in many cultures (both Western and non-Western), and made possible by a staggering range of new technologies, is a case in point. However, these external trends, which particularly impinge on internal processes, should not be taken for granted and can at least become a subject of enquiry and exploration also within our consulting room.

The fate of the body in virtual space

When the narrator in William Gibson's *Neuromancer* starkly pronounced that the body is "data made flesh", he captured the post-human ideal: embodiment is the instantiation of thought. The denial of embodiment emerges as a strong current in discussions about cyberspace and the so-called post-human subject.

Here the "body is the original prosthesis we all learn to manipulate" (Hayles, 1999: 3) and it then becomes possible to add an infinite number of prostheses defying the limits of the given body.

Just as the invention of the car extended the human foot as a prosthesis, technology fundamentally changes us and our experience of our bodies, and hence of our selves as we interact with it. This is vividly captured in the words of one user as he describes his relationship with the computer and the simulated games he played on it:

> When I was away from the machine, I felt as though I had undergone some kind of terminal amputation. With this ability to dislocate functions of my body, with the mediation of my senses, and with this new prosthetic that allowed me to move to another place, I had stepped across a mysterious and fateful line.
>
> (Meadows, 2008: 95)

The "mysterious and fateful line" that can be crossed in virtual reality is deeply seductive. Yet the rate of technological advances far outstrips the mind's capacity to reconcile the triumph of progress with the pain of the inevitable limitations of reality – and especially of our embodied nature. As nature is "transformed into a field of human action" (Giddens, 1991), we have seemingly been freed from the idea that birth is destiny and believe that we can redesign ourselves at will. Many of the developments in cyberspace technology can feed such an illusion.

We are not suggesting that science and technology is a 'bad' thing, but like all good things they can be put to 'bad' use. More specifically, technology de-abjectifies the human body, banishing the messy, internal body and its expelled or leaked fluids. It creates distance from our organic nature and limitations, protecting us from the crude reality, as Becker (1973) provocatively put it, that we are "Gods with anuses". From the point of view of the internal world, avatars, for example, are pseudo-representations of a pseudo-self. For some young people they provide compelling visions of a more desirable self and conveniently bypass what would be a far less certain, messy and painful psychic journey. The way the reality of the body and its psychic meaning can be manipulated in cyberspace is a theme explored by both Lemma and Bonaminio (this edition) in relation to work with adolescents.

The juxtaposition of the 'real' fleshy body in front of a 'hard' computer or a BlackBerry invites pause for thought. Here the complexity of the relationship to the computer as an object of empowerment – its phallic 'hardness' – is exposed through the stark contrast with the softer and folded form of its static user whose body recedes in significance until it becomes superfluous in a virtual world that promises freedom from the constraints of the bodily self.

Focusing on virtual reality, and hence on virtual connectedness, raises the important question of the fate of the body in the mind as the very experience of intimacy because virtual reality is a form of communication that is predicated on distance and a disembodied self. Anzieu (1990) has compellingly argued that today it is no longer sexuality that is repressed; rather, it is the sensual body, the body that comes into being through the other, the body that is denied by technology. The Internet – a wondrous medium for communication – nevertheless has some potentially undesirable psychic implications because it:

> modifies in an entirely new way the feeling of isolation characteristic of each member of the human species; as a result, one's relationship with oneself and the way in which one's internal mental life is cathected are also modified.
>
> (Guignard, 2008: 121)

Just as technological advances promote the *necessity* of digital networks, and "the circulatory systems of flesh and blood are now relegated as merely accessories of bygone times" (Heartney, 2004: 240), so a real relationship to the body, the self and with others can be opted in and out of with ever greater ease. While communication between adolescents through texts and emails may superficially give the impression of close and intimate exchanges, in those young people for whom the body is felt to be terrifying, this virtual intimacy[7] may paradoxically alienate them further from the reality of being-in-a-body. This may create greater difficulties in integrating the sensual and sexual body into a stable self-representation and into meaningful relationships with others.

Indeed, while this vast array of connections has enabled increasingly faster and more efficient communication between individuals and groups of individuals in general, it has also encouraged some individuals to shun real 'human contact' and to connect with a world of 'virtual contacts' instead, or to search for contacts in order to satisfy their perverse conditions. In her chapter, Heather Wood attempts to make sense of compulsive online behaviour and compulsive access to child pornography in particular, which has become an expanding "new phenomenon" and has led to "a growing demand to treat" such Internet offenders.

Psychoanalysis and psychoanalytic interventions in virtual space: encounter, retreat or a helpful bridge to face-to-face contact?

It would be a mistake to only focus on the potential of new technologies to foster pseudo-intimacy. New technologies may also act as catalysts for social relationships, no different in their potential for binding people together than stories or bulletin boards (see Bingham, 1996). For example, one of us (AL) has facilitated two online therapeutic groups, through an online therapeutic community called Big White Wall (see also Graham, 2012). These groups are rooted in psychodynamic ideas both in terms of their content and in the thinking about the therapist's function in the group. The participants were physically located across several different continents, but came together in a closed group for a set number of sessions (set at eight for this pilot study). Needless to say, for a psychoanalyst, this at first felt like a step too far away from psychoanalytic practice, and yet, like any new venture, once the analytic superego could be kept in check, this applied experience turned out to be very instructive and moving. Importantly the intervention also appeared to help people with their experience of depression and anxiety, which had motivated the initial referral to the group (Lemma & Fonagy, in press).

The individuals who joined the group were people who struggled to access mental health services and who were experiencing relatively high levels of distress, typically of an interpersonal nature. The group exchanges were non-synchronous, that is, there was a time delay between postings and response. This was an important feature of the group simultaneously exposing the participants to the frustration of the immediacy typically characteristic of virtual exchanges *and* the containment provided by a therapeutic frame that supported space for reflection.

Over the course of the group, the participants developed important insights into a recurrent, often unconscious, relational pattern that was undermining of their relationships (Lemma, Target & Fonagy, 2011). This pattern was discussed online, and at times enacted through the online interactions with the other group members and/or with the facilitator, which were then commented on by the facilitator. In other words, the transference was live and could be used to shed light on the patterns the participants were working on.

It is beyond the scope of this chapter to enter into a detailed discussion of this way of working and the implications for analytic technique. The main point we want to make is that the sense of community that was engendered by the group process, and the support that participants offered each other, was as 'real' and as significant in its import for the well-being of its individual members, as any group process mobilised in traditional face-to-face group analytic therapy. By the end of both groups, participants reported that they had made important gains in insight and in how they were managing their lives, with some able to take the step to seeking face-to-face therapeutic help.

Such interventions, while departing dramatically from well-trodden psychoanalytic terrain, may yet turn out to be helpful stepping-stones towards therapeutic help for some individuals who would not otherwise avail themselves of help they desperately need. Despite the virtual nature of the medium through which they access help, we are suggesting that a therapeutic process informed by psychoanalytic principles enables such individuals to approach reality in due course rather than representing a defensive retreat away from reality. For example, one participant, who had barely left his room for the preceding three years because he felt anxious and ashamed of himself, and who had managed to approach his local service for face-to-face therapy by the time the group ended, summed up what they had gained from the group thus:

> I've enjoyed having the closer interaction with a smaller group of people. It has certainly helped me to open up a bit more than usual. I think I can see an improvement in opening up and being honest with people about things rather than bottling them up. I think I try to think more rather than rushing in with a response. The biggest thing I think I've learnt here is that the problems I have are not my fault or anyone else's. I still don't like myself much as a person but I think that I don't hate myself like I did before.

While this intervention is psychoanalytically informed it is clearly not psychoanalysis. However, there are now enough people worldwide receiving Skype/telephone psychoanalysis for us to start to explore the benefits and limitations of working in this way as psychoanalysts, both intensively and less intensively.

We are not advocating that online interventions should substitute longer term psychoanalytic psychotherapy or psychoanalysis offered face-to-face; rather, we are suggesting that they may (a) increase accessibility to psychoanalytic treatment, and (b) for a minority of individuals who would find face-to-face therapy/analysis too threatening to begin with, brief psychoanalytically-informed online interventions may provide helpful 'bridges' to accessing face-to-face help.

Communication technology and the analytic setting

Technologies cannot be considered in isolation from the "landscapes of translation" (Wakeford, 1999) in which they are embedded, including when they are used within the analytic setting itself. As various communication systems have altered the way we communicate with each other, they inevitably and perhaps more silently and subtly have also permeated the psychoanalytic setting. However, we still don't really know how they have affected it. Have they changed the way we work? Have they really forged a new form of communication? Have they intruded on or complemented the analytic setting, which by definition relies on the subtle nuances of language, observation and a number of other sensorial experiences that are time-honoured instruments of the psychoanalytic profession?

Gabbard (this edition) helps us to establish an ongoing dialogue about unfamiliar and creative ways of communicating with patients by bringing email communication into the boundary of the analytic space and questioning its unique properties including "a playful expansion of the self ... [and] of the analytic experience". Scharff (this edition) and Sabbadini (this edition) extend this discussion by exploring the particular setting of telephone and Skype analysis and how the analyst can manage this so as to preserve the analytic attitude. While this virtual setting undoubtedly impacts on both analyst and patient, and introduces an additional dimension to the therapeutic relationship that requires analysis, the analyst doing telenalysis is no different to an analyst who works with his patients in the actual consulting room.

The development of psychoanalysis in countries such as Russia, China and Japan has been facilitated by new technologies allowing training analyses to take place. These are important developments for psychoanalysis as a discipline and could not have taken place without the assistance of these new technologies. We might well ask, of course, 'but at what cost?' Indeed, we need to seriously consider to what extent teleanalysis or Skype analysis can represent a good enough form of training analysis for candidates. Scharff (this edition) aptly questions whether we can consider it as:

> functionally equivalent to an in-person analysis in terms of fostering dreaming, free association, resistance, and transference-countertransference experience of sufficient intensity to evoke in candidates having teleanalysis a conviction about the working of the unconscious, the formation of character defenses, and the interpretive skill to achieve therapeutic action such that these candidates become effective analysts with their own analysands.
>
> (p. 59)

This remains an important question that the new generations of analysts trained in this manner will hopefully help us to better understand. Moreover there may be important distinctions even between a telephone analysis and a Skype analysis whereby the actual form of technology that facilitates the disembodied contact between the analytic couple will expose the patient to different frustrations and/or gratifications, which will acquire idiosyncratic significance in the transference.

The opportunity to have an analysis by Skype or telephone where there is no other option because of vast geographical distances has supported the more widespread provision of psychoanalysis and not only for training purposes. Sabbadini (this edition), however, questions another emergent phenomenon, namely those patients who can manage to come to their sessions in person but opt not to. Here Skype analysis might well be regarded as another form of resistance rather than a necessary modification of the analytic setting in the service of providing analysis where there would otherwise be none available. Given that virtual communication is present nowadays in so many areas of life – 'the way things are' – there is a risk for the analyst of being drawn into agreeing to such arrangements when they are presented by the patient as part and parcel of what we all do.

When considering the meaning of reality as opposed to virtual reality, we cannot deny that what we call the conventional analytic setting is in itself a curious and unusual combination of real and artificial reality. The analytic setting, along with the analytic attitude, creates a space that is as unique as it is at odds with many other social and professional encounters. Most human relationships unfold in contexts that are not timed to the very last minute and where shaking each other's hand or yielding to phatic communication smooth social interaction rather than potentially become the focus for a discussion of unconscious processes. Even professional and boundaried relationships such as those with medical practitioners do not approximate the 'oddness' of the analytic situation.

The standard analytic frame commonly relies on the actual presence of the analyst and patient, a chair and a couch along with the remaining furnishing of the consulting room and may include the waiting area. In addition, the act of "getting to the analyst and the analytic room", the physical holding of the analytic room in the real presence of the analyst, along with sharing the same common physical reality of the here and now represent important "transitions" (Lin, 2011) enabling both analyst and patient to gradually build and make contact with one another.

This long established, but still 'unusual', setting lends itself to the development of a special space between analyst and patient. It is within the safety of this unique space that a mutually agreed interaction takes place while a trusting relationship is gradually built promoting the unfolding of a narrative and reverie – accompanied by curiosity, imagination and fantasy. Moreover this interaction is imbued with a gamut of emotional conscious and unconscious communications, both in the analyst and patient. Both verbal and non-verbal sensory-motor nuances along with the affective undertones are thus in a constant interplay. The lying on the couch, away from the analyst's gaze may favour this interaction – or may indeed thwart it, particularly in sensitive and severely disturbed patients – by freeing both the analyst and the patient from their mutual visual exposure. Paradoxically, it is through this very absence of visual stimulation that the perception of other senses can be enhanced (or at times even diminished) while giving way to more unconscious processes during this unique process of reflecting. Among some of the non-verbal communications, silence coupled with the absence of the visual component, for example, can occupy a significant and meaningful space, the origin of which can be analysed and eventually understood. At other times a body posture, gestures, peculiar movements or a certain gaze can convey a highly specific affective communication, which may be in keeping or totally at odds with the actual verbal component. In other words, the common reality of an ordinary encounter is partially suspended in order to create this new artificial physical and metaphorical space – a kind of virtual space that exists within a particular time frame: after 50 minutes that frame is 'switched off', much like one might turn the computer off as the patient leaves the room and re-engages with their ongoing reality.

It goes without saying that these subtleties, among many others, may be distorted or not captured at all when the patient's (and analyst's) body is absent from the real analytic room. For example, as silence can be perceived differently in the absence of bodily presence in these forms of communication, it is not uncommon to find ourselves being more talkative with patients over the phone (Bassen, 2007), perhaps because the sense of cut-offness is often starker than in the actual consulting room.

Another cornerstone of the analytic setting has been the preservation of privacy through the maintenance of the so-called 'blank screen' held by the analyst. This 'spurious' anonymity is advocated in order to foster, and subsequently analyse, the onset of fantasies about the analyst in the patient, which may then be traced back to the patient's narrative and 're-examined' within the transference and counter-transference responses. While analysts will probably continue to struggle between the needs for privacy and self-disclosure (Kantrowitz, 2007), generally speaking patients tend to respect their analyst's private life, while their curiosity is usually confined to the analyst's moods and thoughts within the consulting room. Moreover patients may glean more information about the analyst's origin, culture, qualifications, personal taste and so on from a number of sources including the analyst's accent, use of words, clothing style and type of furnishing of the consulting room. If this is not enough, they may satisfy their curiosity through other means, for example, the analyst's writings, lectures, conferences or other encounters outside the analytic room. All this, if and when brought to the surface, is generally deemed to be 'good material to analyse'.

However, with the advent of the Internet and other forms of media communication we have to come to terms with the fact that curiosity will be satisfied through other means. As Gabbard forcefully declared during an international panel on virtual reality: "The classical view of psychoanalytic anonymity is dead!"; hence we have to resign ourselves to the fact that privacy has now become a temporary phenomenon (Vinocur Fischbein, 2010). Cyberspace has thus inevitably rendered the space between the public and private sphere rather thin and therefore we can now assume that our 'anonymous' identity as ordinary people as well as psychoanalysts is 'doomed to disappear online'. We need to work with its implications within the analytic relationship and to conceptualise the way the changing external context impinges or alters the classical analytic setting. For example, as texts become the primary means of communication for adolescents, and indeed also for many adults, many mental health services have moved to using this as the main means of communication between the clinic and the patient. This kind of standardisation of a virtual means of communication that is very immediate and less 'formal' even than a telephone message, no doubt may be used defensively by some adolescent patients, but we can no longer simply view it as a deviation from the analytic setting; rather it is the classical analytic setting that has been modified to accommodate changing patterns of communication in our society.

Of course, the use made of technology in the analytic setting deserves our continued psychoanalytic curiosity and analysis as it impacts on the analytic couple. While in ordinary analysis the control of the analytic setting remains largely in the hands of the analyst in that the basic 'one way' rules are clearly established by the analyst from the outset, in teleanalysis and other forms of communication such as telephone, emails or texts, its responsibility tends to be shared between the analyst and the patient in a more concrete way. They require in addition the actual presence, familiarity and mutually agreed exchange of these new technologies needing to be regularly switched on and charged or repaired when necessary. For example, a number of disappointments may occur with the use of Skype and it may well be necessary to clarify from the outset that there may be persistent problems with interruptions and line connection, with the quality of sound and the clarity of visual contact achieved on screen. Such eventualities can threaten stability and generate a certain amount of extra anxiety in the patient, as well as in the analyst, which needs to be taken into account. However, it could be argued that unpredictability is part and parcel of life and therefore also of any analytic setting. The meaning ascribed to these technological difficulties by both patient and analyst can provide useful material for discussion.

As we will see in this book, for some patients cyberspace has clearly created a 'new extra object' with the attached risk of becoming all encompassing, and it makes them highly dependent on it. At other times, however, for some patients, it is used as a vital bridge, or as a buffer, in an attempt to maintain continuity with the analyst and in that way offsets the threat of sudden separation, abandonment and loneliness. For example, a patient (of LC) whose fragmented state of mind could be barely contained in her three weekly sessions, often left text messages on the answering machine in between sessions in order to communicate her distress including her self-harm and suicidal ideation. Although the analyst hardly responded, she also often expressed her gratitude for having the opportunity to maintain continuity with her analyst through this means.

If it is clear that special circumstances may warrant a modification and incorporation of new technologies in the analytic setting. After carefully ascertaining the reasons for them, we may have to be flexible and adapt our way of working according to the needs of our patients, provided that *our analytic listening remains the most valuable tool guiding our work*. Communication technology and the analytic setting can mix and work in harmony as long as the process between analyst and patient remains a central focus and modifications to the setting are monitored for their unconscious meaning and psychic functions.

Conclusions

At this point in time, can we state that the cyberspace has changed our overall mode of communication and has impinged on our psychoanalytic practice? No doubt it has inevitably intermingled in our lives as psychoanalytic practitioners and has posed a challenge to a number of our psychoanalytic assumptions, most importantly in relation to the analytic setting and frame.

Perhaps not enough time has gone by in order to obtain a clearer picture about the use of cyberspace in psychoanalytic circles. It could be argued, however, that this is because any pace of change in the psychoanalytic world takes too long or it may even have to occur 'secretly' before unusual or unconventional methods of working become common knowledge and thus influence or are endorsed in our clinical practice. As it is well known, any innovation by definition inevitably attracts both acolytes and detractors and the same applies to the psychoanalytic world. Hence, more psychoanalysts and psychoanalytic practitioners will have to experiment with these communication systems, often under special or unusual circumstances and 'put their head above the parapet' by being curious and candid about some of these new ways of working so that we can evaluate them without prejudice.

Notes

1 A software application making use of phone calls and video conferencing over the Internet.
2 Partly or entirely replacing face-to-face contact.
3 The provision of personalised health care over a distance for severe chronic conditions such as problematic asthmatic, diabetic and HIV patients.
4 Strong links are those constituted by family and close friends as opposed to more casual and unplanned brief contacts in weak links.
5 A publicly accessible journal maintained on the web by an individual or a group and inviting comments and debates online.
6 A vulnerable patient suffering from identity issues and depression (LC), who indulged in 'chats on line' in order to form 'meaningful relationships' was regularly disappointed and rejected when the 'real encounters' did not match his fantasy and expectations. Indeed these individuals turned out to be even more vulnerable than he was.
7 Sigman (2009) has drawn attention to the potentially deleterious impact of social networking sites on both relationships and possibly even on biology.

References

Anzieu, D. (1990) *A Skin for Thought: Interviews with Gilbert Tarrab on Psychology and Psychoanalysis*. London: Karnac.

Bassen, C. (2007) Telephone Analysis. *Journal of the American Psychoanalytic Association* 55: 1033–1041.

Baudrillard, J. (1996) *The Perfect Crime*. London: Verso.

Becker, E. (1973) *The Denial of Death*. New York: Free Press.
Bingham, N. (1996) Objections: From Technological Determinism Towards Geographies of Relations. *Society and Space 15*(6): 635–657.
Bingham, N. (1999) Unthinkable Complexity: Cyberspace Otherwise. In: M. Crang, P. Crang and J. May (Eds) *Virtual Geographies*. London: Routledge.
Bion, W. R. (1961) *Experiences in Groups*. London: Tavistock Publications.
Bonaminio, V. (2010) See under Vinocur Fischbein.
Carlino, R. (2010) *Distance Psychoanalysis*. London: Karnac.
Chartier, R. (1997) *On the Edge of the Cliff: History, Language, Practices*. Baltimore, MD: John Hopkins University Press.
Cohen, A. (2001) Visual Hollywood and the Genealogy of Its Hyper-Spectator. In: M. Stokes and R. Maltby (Eds) *Hollywood Spectatorship*. London: British Film Institute.
Cohen, B. (1996) *The Edge of Chaos: Financial Booms, Bubbles and Crashes*. New York: Wiley.
Daintith, J. (2008) *Oxford Dictionary of Computing*. Oxford: Oxford University Press.
Delueze, G. (1994) *Difference and Repetition*. London: Athlone.
Dini, K. (2009) Internet Interaction: The Effects on Patient's Lives and Analytic Process. *Journal of the American Psychoanalytic Association* 57: 979–988.
Doel, M. and Clarke, B. (2006) Virtual Worlds: Suppletion, S(ed)uction and Simulacra. In: M. Crang, P. Crang and J. May (Eds) *Virtual Geographies*. London: Routledge.
Ermann, M. (2004) On Medial Identity. *International Forum of Psychoanalysis 13*: 275–283.
Fink, J. (1999). *Cyberseduction: Reality in the Age of Psychotechnology*. Amherst, NY: Prometheus Books.
Fiorentini, G. (2011) L'Analisi Via Internet: Variazioni di Setting e Dinamiche Transferali-Controtransferali. Paper presented at Centro Milanese di Psicoanalisi Cesare Musatti.
Fischer, C. (2007) Technology and Community: Historical Complexities. *Sociological Inquiry* 67(1): 113–118.
Fornari-Spoto, G. (2011) *Bulletin of the British Psychoanalytical Society* 47: 7–11.
Gibson, W. (1984) *Neuromancer*. New York: Ace Books.
Giddens, A. (1991) *Modernity and Self Identity*. Cambridge: Polity.
Graham, R. (2012) Where Internet Was, There Ego Shall Be: Community and Well-Being in the Digital World. In: A. Lemma (Ed.) *Contemporary Developments in Adult and Young Adult Therapy: The Work of the Tavistock and Portman Clinics*. London: Karnac.
Guignard, S. (2008) Envy in Western Society: Today and Tomorrow. In: P. Roth and A. Lemma (Eds) *Envy and Gratitude Revisited*. London: Karnac.
Hayles, C. (1999) *How We Became Posthuman*. Chicago: Chicago University Press.
Hayles, N. (1993) Virtual Bodies and Flickering Signifiers. *October* 66: 69–91.
Heartney, E. (2004) Orlan: Magnificent 'and' Best. In: R. Durand and E. Heartney (Eds) *Orlan: Carnal Art*. Paris: Flammarion.
Heim, M. (1998) *Virtual Realism*. New York: Oxford University Press.
Herzfeld, M. (1992) *The Social Production of Indifference*. Chicago: University of Chicago Press.
Hillis, K. (1999). *Digital Sensations: Space, Identity, and Embodiment in Virtual Reality*. Minneapolis, MN: University of Minnesota Press.

Hofling, C (1979) An Instance of Psychotherapy Continued by Correspondence. *Bulletin of the Menninger Clinic, 43*: 393–412.

Jones, D. (2006) I, Avatar: Constructions of Self and Place in Second Life and the Technological Imagination. *Gnovis, 6*. Available at http:/gnovis journals.org/files/ Donald-e-ones-I-Avatar pdf (accessed 20 December 2011).

Kantrowitz, J. (2007) Privacy and Disclosure in Psychoanalysis. *Journal of the American Psychoanalytic Association 57*: 787–806.

Kilborne, B. (2011) Personal communication.

Koch, R. and Lockwood, G. (2010) *Superconnect. The Power of Networks and the Strength of Weak Links*. London: Little, Brown.

Leffert, M. (2003) Analysis and Psychotherapy by Telephone. *Journal of the American Psychoanalytic Association 51*: 101–130.

Lemma, A. and Fonagy, F. (under review) A Feasibility Study of a Psychodynamic Online Group Intervention for Depression and Anxiety.

Lemma, A., Target, M. and Fonagy, P. (2011) *Dynamic Interpersonal Therapy: A Clinician's Guide*. Oxford: Oxford University Press.

Lin, T. (2011) Skype Analysis: Problems and Limitations. Training paper.

Lindon, J. (1988) Psychoanalysis by Telephone. *Bulletin of the Menninger Clinic 52*: 521–528.

Lindon, J., Lewin, B. D., Ballint, M., Fleming, J., Gill, M., Grinberg, L., Searles, H. F., Josseling, I. M. and Wallerstein, R. S. (1972) Supervision by Tape: A New Method of Case Supervision. *Psychoanalysis Forum 4*: 399–452.

Lingiardi, V. (2008) Playing with Unreality: Transference and Computer. *International Journal of Psychoanalysis 89*: 111–126.

McLean, S., Protti, D. and Sheikh, A. (2011) Telehealth Care for Long Term Conditions. *British Medical Journal 342*: 120.

Meadows, M. (2008) *I, Avatar: The Culture and Consequences of Having a Second Life*. San Francisco, CA: New Riders Press.

Powers, W. (2010) *Hamlet's BlackBerry*. New York: HarperCollins.

Reuters (2011) *Sorry, Catholics Can't Confess Via the New Iphone App*. FaithWorld. Available at http://blogs.reuters.com/faithworld/tag/apps/ (accessed 10 February 2013)

Riva, G. (2005). Virtual Reality in Psychotherapy. *Cyberpsychology and Behaviour 8*(3): 220–230.

Robins, K. (2001) Seeing the World from a Safe Distance. *Science as Culture 10*(4): 531–539.

Rosenbaum, M. (1977) Premature Interruption of Psychotherapy: Continuation of Contact by Telephone and Correspondence. *American Journal of Psychoanalysis 134*: 200–202.

Scharff, J. (2010). Telephone Analysis. Panel report. *International Journal of Psychoanalysis 91*: 989–992.

Sigman, A. (2009) Well Connected? The Biological Implications of Social Networking. *Biologist 56*(1): 14–20.

Steiner, J. (1993) *Psychic Retreats*. London: Routledge.

Stewart, R. S. and Nicholls, R. (2002) Virtual Worlds, Travel, and the Picturesque Garden. *Philosophy and Geography 5*(1): 83–99.

Symington, N. (2011) Analysis and Supervision by Telephone and Skype: Letter. *Bulletin of the British Psychoanalytical Society 47*(9): 46.

Thomson, J. (1995) The *Media and Modernity: A Social Theory of the Media*. Cambridge: Polity Press.
Vinocur Fischbein, S. (2010) Psychoanalysis and Virtual Reality. Panel Report. *International Journal of Psychoanalysis 91*: 985–988.
Wakeford, N. (1999) Gender and the Landscapes of Computing in an Internet Café. In: M. Crang, P. Crang and J. May (Eds) *Virtual Geographies*. London: Routledge.
White, M. (2006) *The Body and the Screen: Theories of Internet Spectatorship*. London: MIT Press.

Chapter 1

New technologies and the psychoanalytic setting

Andrea Sabbadini

Once upon a time, back in the 1970s, bulky answering machines started to expand the range of our telephone facilities. I well remember the resistance of many analysts, myself included, in accepting that such devices could also be useful for exchanging messages with our patients, say about the cancellation of sessions. The debate about the intrusion of technology into our clinical work, centred then on the appropriateness or otherwise of using audio or even video recordings of sessions for training or research purposes, became extended to the one concerning new telephone technologies.

Of course, answering machines, not unlike everything else, could be used for defensive goals, such as in order to avoid a more personal verbal interaction ('If you need to give me a message outside a session, you may at least make the effort to tell me in person!'). From our current perspective, however, such a justification sounds weak, and we can hardly imagine any therapist today objecting to the practice of leaving or receiving voice messages – though such therapists would still want, whenever appropriate, to interpret their patient's motives for using this form of communication – or, indeed, for refusing to do so.

The landline telephones in our consulting rooms, meanwhile, have been to a large extent replaced by mobiles and smartphones, which also offer the facility of exchanging written text messages (in addition to voice ones), now used as a norm between analysts and patients but, again, at first resisted by many colleagues for analogous reasons ('If you need to leave me a message outside a session, you may at least make the effort to do so with your own voice!').

Come the 1980s and many of us began to indulge in the expensive habit of acquiring personal computers. We could not then have predicted, however, the extent to which their development would have eventually affected our professional work – in the area of research with the help of large databases of information, such as PEP and Wikipedia, and of powerful search engines, and in our clinical activities. In particular, the easy and ever-faster access to the Internet since the late 1980s, with its website and email facilities, has revolutionized the way in which we operate as psychoanalysts, the way in which we relate to our patients (and they to us) and, as a corollary, the way in which we conceive of our own professional identity.

Nowadays the impact of new communication technologies is felt by all psychoanalysts and psychotherapists, including those who may be unable or unwilling, for a variety of reasons, to make much use of them. I consider such an impact on our work to be fundamentally positive. Although some aspects of it are a source of concern, for instance the increased difficulty to preserve the confidentiality of clinical material, I believe that those in our profession who object in principle to technological progress, like the Luddites had done in the nineteenth-century textile industry, are self-defeatingly destined to be left behind. But especially in these first decades of the electronic revolution there is a price to be paid, often before we can make available to us the intellectual and emotional resources to pay it.

Software, cyberspace, teleconferencing, laptops, DVD rewriters, digitalization, webcams... In the course of hardly one generation a whole vocabulary has entered our worlds and everybody has had to familiarize him or herself (some more successfully than others, of course) with a vast number of new words, ideas, objects and activities. An enormous, but steadily dwindling, population has thus come into existence of what Prensky (2001) has called 'digital immigrants': those who, myself included, grew up before the new electronic technologies were developed, in contrast with the new generation of 'digital natives', familiar since their childhood with the language of computers, video games and the Internet, and more comfortable than most of us with establishing and maintaining relationships from a distance through social networking sites. Who still remembers having a 'pen friend'?

Such a process has involved a loss of competences, and the need to replace them with alternative ones. Because of the speed of the electronic revolution, these enforced changes and readjustments have often been experienced as traumatic, including by psychoanalysts. A number of unconscious defences, such as denial, have been mobilized to deal with the confusion thus engendered in our sense of professional identity.

That the rapid development and increased availability of such communication technologies is having, for better or worse, a major impact on most aspects of our everyday life is an unquestionable truth. In our work, electronic mails and SMS have to a large extent replaced letters and telephone conversations, making the exchange of ideas and information among colleagues, members of committees and administrators faster and more efficient. At the same time, these media are also being used by patients and analysts to communicate with each other about matters such as the rearrangement of sessions. This may affect the maintenance of analytic boundaries and therefore the nature of our relationship with patients.

About a year ago I received an email from a Mr D. He was asking for a consultation because he had decided, as he put it, 'to embark on an analysis'.

I replied by giving him my mobile telephone number so that he could call me up to make an appointment – which he did. Several SMS from him followed – to change the date of our meeting because he had suddenly decided to take a holiday, to check my address, to confirm the new date of the consultation, etc. Having finally arrived on the right day, at the right time and in the right place, Mr D called me up again from outside my front door to check that the bell he was going to ring was the right one.

In the course of the consultation Mr D confessed that he had already 'Googled me up' and was pleased to have discovered that I had published articles on cinema and psychoanalysis as he had himself a great interest in films. He also informed me that he would be available to attend only one weekly session, something that I explained I was not prepared to do as I see my patients more frequently. Mr D insisted it was me he wanted to see. As I could not comply with his request I referred him to a colleague – something which, feeling rejected by me, he only reluctantly accepted.

A week later I received an email from Mr D with a link to a website: the advertisement of a company offering discounted Viagra, Cialis and other such pharmaceutical products. Having overcome my initial surprise (and, I must add, considerable annoyance), I reasoned that Mr D must have felt powerless to obtain from me what he wanted ('embarking on an analysis') and projected his own impotence onto me, to then present me with a cheap chemical solution to 'my' problem.

The reason why I am reporting this vignette is to make the point that none of this – contacting me by email, leaving SMS texts, checking my credentials on Google, sending me a link to an Internet website – could have happened only a few years ago.

My specific concern in this chapter is about the impact of new communication technologies on the psychoanalytic setting and, in turn, about how such an impact may affect our analytic attitude and, more generally, our analytic identity.

I will consider here what changes to our classic setting are required to allow psychoanalytic supervision or therapeutic sessions to be carried out with the help of electronic devices; how our attitude towards supervisees and patients may be altered by such changes; and how our own sense of who we are (what we believe in, and what, why and how we do it) is influenced as a result – to such an extent, perhaps, that our analytic identity may end up being transformed also when we happen to resume working in our usual, more conventional ways.

For many years now psychoanalysts have been engaging in telephone supervision and analysis (Bassen 2007; Leffert 2003; Zalusky 2003). At first this was done in order to deal with the problem of candidates living too far away from any training analysts to be able to attend sessions in person, sometimes because a recognized psychoanalytic society did not exist yet in their own countries; the only way for these candidates to train was therefore to do so from a distance, i.e. over the telephone. This practice, sometimes referred to as 'teleanalysis' (Scharff 2010 and this edition) or 'distance analysis' (Carlino 2010), was extended to situations where either patient or analyst had to move abroad or to a different city for work or family reasons (a development made more impelling by the increasingly frequent phenomenon of geographical mobility) and the only way for the analysis, originally taking place in the consulting room, to continue was to conduct it over the telephone. In these cases, sometimes the analyst recommended that meetings in person would also take place, if only sporadically, for the two participants in the analytic couple to remind themselves of what it feels like to share the same physical space. On a more short-term basis, telephone meetings would replace the more conventional ones when patients undergoing analysis became affected by an illness or had to move temporarily to a far-away place for work reasons, thus being prevented to attend their sessions in person.

All these situations have persisted over time and, from what I can infer from the relevant literature and from informal conversations with colleagues, have in fact become more frequent as well as acceptable to a growing number of practitioners. In the last few years, though, distance psychoanalysis has been spreading also as a result of choice rather than necessity, with patients opting for meeting in cyberspace even when they could have easily done so in the consulting room – a questionable practice because of the likelihood that its main purpose is to circumvent resistance to the in-person analytic process. In other words it is not invariably so, but we need to remain open to the possibility that it is being used as a form of resistance.

The ever-more common practice to conduct psychoanalytic and supervision sessions over the telephone, or even by email (see Gabbard, this edition; Carlino 2010), has been a source of considerable debate. Some authors would claim that 'the present state of modern telecommunications … must be taken as a new opportunity to allow for the implementation of analysis beyond the walls of the psychoanalyst's office' (Carlino 2010, p. 3), thus much increasing its accessibility. Others would find it 'difficult to accept the argument that psychoanalysis, or we psychoanalysts, have to chase after the changing times and society. Our task', they point out, 'is to understand and interpret change' (Argentieri & Amati Mehler, 2003, p. 18).

I shall limit myself here to explore some of the implications for the analytic setting, attitude and identity of sessions carried out by such video-links as Skype: a more sophisticated means of communication than the telephone, more compatible with our conventional ways of practicing psychoanalysis and, besides, more likely for these reasons to become widespread. I shall introduce the neologism 'skypanalyis' to refer to such practice.

As most readers probably know, Skype is the video conferencing software programme that allows those engaging in conversation to also watch each other on their respective computer screens. Importantly, Skype also shows your own image in a corner of the screen: a small mirror, in effect, which may acquire special significance in the context of the therapeutic setting where normally, in the absence of mirrors, people cannot see themselves.

It must be said that Skype technology, at least in its present state, is far from flawless: for instance, the sound of the voices may become distorted or lose its synchronicity with the images, and the video may at times freeze. Furthermore, if in the course of a session the Internet connection on either side gets interrupted, the communication (and therefore the session) is also discontinued – a frustrating and not infrequent occurrence. Which fantasies are then likely to be activated? Was the interruption deliberate? Will it be restored, and if so when? What changes to the setting should be brought about to deal with it? Should the time that had been missed out for analytic work during the interruption be made up at the end of the session for it to have lasted its full 50 minutes?

Related to these issues, at least as far as the fantasies that could be evoked are concerned, is the often-encountered occurrence of silences in the course of a session. When the two participants in the analytic couple communicate from a distance, silence on either side can feel more difficult to tolerate than it would if they were in the same room. This is because silence, especially when visual contact is not available, may be experienced as threatening, making it more likely to get broken prematurely in an attempt to prevent the emergence of anxieties of abandonment or persecution. These can take the form of paranoid fantasies such as doubts about whether the other person is really being silent, or if the analysis is being carried out by telephone, that the analyst has instead left the room, got distracted doing something else, or even perhaps dropped dead. Poland pointed out that patients in his office 'sometimes ask "Are you asleep?" but on the phone they ask "Are you there?"' (quoted by Bassen 2007, p. 1034).

Another consideration is that, unlike in sessions taking place in a consulting room, during video-calls the bodies of the two participants only share a virtual space, also known as cyberspace. There is no doubt that the physical presence of the analyst's and the analysand's bodies plays an important part in their interaction, with repercussions on the transference and counter-transference. Is it then possible to thus dispose of bodies, or rather of their actual presence in a physical space, without this having major implications on the analytic process? How will their absence alter the quality of the communication between the analytic couple – indeed, any couple?

It is true that patients using the couch have only a few brief moments to look at their analysts at the beginning and the end of sessions, and analysts sitting in a chair behind their patients only have limited visual access to their bodies. It is also true that physical contact between them is mostly non-existent, and that other perceptual modalities (such as smell) only rarely come to play a significant part in the analytic relationship. However, the mere *possibility* of, say, bodily contact between them, be it of an erotic, affectionate or aggressive nature, is central to the experience (both actual and transferential) that therapist and patient have of each other. The absence of such possibility in skypanalysis, therefore, is not a matter of indifference.

We may add that although in the virtual space of distant analysis the two bodies of analyst and patient are not simultaneously present in the same location, we now have to factor in a third presence replacing, as well as representing, them: that of the electronic machinery (computers with their microphones and cameras), which at least in the first few sessions, before those using them get accustomed to it, cannot but disturb the intimacy and privacy of the analytic relationship. This interference will often have all sorts of connotations, including in the area of Oedipal fantasies, possibly stimulating curiosity, jealousy and persecutory anxieties. None of this, it could be argued, is a bad thing in itself, but it does require careful handling and interpretation. In this respect Yamin Habib comments that:

> the analyst's acceptance of the involvement of a permanent third party in the relationship – even if the third party is an instrument – modifies the conventional setting so drastically that it is appropriate to consider whether the resulting process diverges substantially from *psychoanalysis as such*.
>
> (2003, p. 26, my emphasis)

The answer to this question, it seems to me, depends on our definition of 'psychoanalysis as such'.

Should the conventional analytic setting of couch and armchair be somehow replicated when sessions occur by video-call? Should skypanalysis be set up in an asymmetrical way, so that the camera is only switched on in the patient's room (allowing the analyst to see him), but not in the therapist's? The analyst would then be sitting in his/her consulting room's chair with her laptop in front of her showing her analysand on the screen, while the patient would be lying down on a couch in his own home, analogously as he would have done if he were in the actual presence of his therapist, perhaps with the webcam placed behind his head to give the analyst a similarly limited view of him. Such an artificial setting, mimicking the more usual analytic one, can easily lead to distortions in transference and counter-transference dynamics. A preferable arrangement would be for therapist and patient engaged in skypanalysis is to sit in front of their computers with both webcams switched on, thus reproducing the face-to-face setting – not an ideal arrangement, of course, but perhaps a worthy compromise if it allows psychoanalysis to take place at all between participants otherwise living too far from each other to meet in person on a frequent basis.

It is crucial to acknowledge that relationships and communication taking place in a physical space are fundamentally different from those happening in cyberspace. Any denial of such differences and attempts to reproduce the classic setting in the kind of virtual reality where distant sessions occur are doomed to failure. For instance, the importance of the temporal dimension in psychoanalysis, and the peculiar coexistence of its timeless quality with the presence of rigorous time boundaries (Sabbadini 1989) is even more prominent in skypanalysis: this is because the same 50-minute time shared by the two protagonists on such a psychoanalytic stage replaces, so to speak, the physical space they would have occupied had they engaged in classic analysis. As Carlino notices, a feature of distance analysis is that 'analytic dialogue ... is measured from communicational parameters of time ... and not in patterns of geographic distance measured in the metric system' (2010, p. 64).

On the other hand, the assumption that only the conventional way of carrying out analysis is the 'correct' one, and the one most likely to bring positive therapeutic results simply because it is what we are used to, is questionable. In her report on a panel held at a recent IPA congress, Savege Scharff wrote about teleanalysis: 'psychoanalysis is primarily the encounter with an understanding mind *in whatever setting that may occur*' (2010, p. 990, my emphasis). The evidence built on over a century of psychoanalytic experience suggests that changes to the original setting, as long as they respect certain basic technical and ethical parameters, can be advantageous to both analysts and patients, should be welcome whenever their enforcement improves the quality of the work and are anyway inevitable as the external environment (which, in our case, includes the widespread presence of electronic technologies in all aspects of life) evolves.

Freud (1912), who had described his technical principles for carrying out analytic work, was the first to concede that these were not fixed and should be constantly reviewed; indeed he had called them 'recommendations'. Consistent with this tolerant approach, in the course of his own life-time Freud had replaced hypnotherapy with the free associative method and had discontinued the holding of his hand on the patient's forehead; the habit of fixing a date for termination had given way to open-ended analysis, the norm of six weekly sessions was reduced to five; and so on.

A source of concern in the electronic age relates to our wish to preserve analytic privacy, anonymity and neutrality. While adherence to abstinence (defined as the principle that those desires expressed in the course of psychoanalysis should always be interpreted rather than acted upon) remains paramount in our practice; the fantasy that we could maintain anonymity has always been the result of unrealistic wishful thinking. It is every analyst's experience to feel amazed by how accurately some patients seem to 'know' us, or indeed how far from the truth they could be (one of my patients, who knew about my Italian origins, was convinced that I was the son of the Pope!).

More recently, new communication technologies have wide-opened the access to information about others, analysts included. Many patients nowadays, as in the vignette I have reported above, would 'Google up' their therapists' name and find all pieces of information, some of it inaccurate, about them. This, in Gabbard's words, 'has hammered the nails in the coffin of analytic anonymity' (quoted by Vinocur Fishbein 2010, p. 986). We should then accept that our wish for privacy, anonymity and, as a consequence also neutrality, cannot be sustained. Such realization, of course, should never prevent us from interpreting whenever appropriate the patient's curiosity about us.

For what concerns the setting, distance analysis, not unlike classic analysis, would require the rigorous preservation of constancy and consistency. The analytic contract, preferably stipulated in the course of an initial in-person interview in the consulting room of the psychoanalyst, should specify not only such details as the amount and form of payment of fees, but also that sessions take place at regular times and intervals, and with both analyst and analysand engaging in telecommunication with each other from a constant location, e.g. sitting for every session in the same room, thus replicating the face-to-face configuration, rather than the couch-and-armchair one. Mutual trust from both participants is essential for the implementation of such basic rules.

It is also worth noticing that the communication tools needed by both participants for engaging in distance analysis (computers, webcams, Internet connection, Skype software, etc.) and the activities required for activating them (such as ensuring to be online, and for the analysand to make the call at the agreed-upon time) all become part of the new setting; as such, both their presence and the ways in which they are being utilized are likely to affect transference and counter-transference dynamics, and therefore become a potential focus of interpretations. The boundaries surrounding this virtual setting are inevitably different from those present in physical space, even if their main function of protecting the analysis from external intrusions remains the same.

As far as their sense of professional identity is concerned, psychoanalysts are likely to experience an initial feeling of dislocation when they start practicing from a virtual space, similarly perhaps to the one they would feel if they were to move their practice to a different consulting room; this, however, should subside as the analysis progresses and both participants get accustomed to the new setting. After all, whether we meet our analysands in a consulting room or in cyberspace, we are still psychoanalysts engaged in the psychoanalytic process; we are still committed to making a safe environment (the setting) available to our patients, where we empathetically listen in a state of suspended attention to their free associations. This material will consist of mostly verbal (but also para-verbal and extra-verbal), emotionally-loaded communications: memories of past events, reports of recent ones, unconscious fantasies and daydreams, feelings and observations about the here-and-now of the analytic situation, wishes and fears, future plans, dreams and nightmares. Analysts seeing their patients on Skype will relate to this material in a similar way and with a similar attitude as they would if the patients were physically present in their consulting rooms. This involves, whenever appropriate, suggesting links among different parts of the material and providing interpretations that would take into account such issues as resistance and defensive mechanisms, internal conflictual configurations, as well as the transferential and counter-transferential aspects of the analytic relationship. The rituals surrounding the analytic meetings may be different (e.g. going to the consulting room and ringing the doorbell versus going online and making a video-call), but not the substance itself of the psychoanalytic process (see also Scharff, this edition).

It seems to me that the question to be asked in this context is not whether analyst and patient should ever agree to meet in the virtual space of the Internet rather than in the physical one of the consulting room in those situations when the latter is unreachable to the patient. Whether we approve of it or not, this is already happening on a large scale, even if analysts rarely talk about it with colleagues – perhaps because of 'their unanalysed guilt over transgressing traditional psychoanalytic norms' (Zalusky 2003, p. 16). The few systematic surveys to date (e.g Fornari-Spoto 2011) suggest that about one-third of psychoanalysts have at least experimented with distant analysis, and that the increase in the proportion of such practices parallels the growth of the population of digital natives among analysts and patients. However, no proper statistics are available about the actual number of analyses or supervisions carried out in this form, or about the reasons given for selecting such a modality.

The important issue here is whether the simultaneous presence of the analytic dyad in a physical space is a condition *sine qua non* for the psychoanalytic process to occur. It could be argued that it is, on the grounds that the emotional aspect of human relationships can only properly find expression in such a context. But it could also be argued that facilities such as video-links (unlike emails, which convey only written words, or the telephone, which transmits only sounds) do in fact provide the main perceptual features, visual and auditory, for meaningful communication. Traditional physical analytic encounters may still be preferable to virtual ones, but they would not constitute a necessary condition for the analytic process to unfold and for effective therapeutic work to occur.

Some may question whether sessions carried out on the Internet could still be described as being psychoanalytic ones, considering the changes thus imposed upon the traditional setting and the implications this could have for our analytic professional identity. The answer to this question, of course, depends on how rigid (as different from rigorous) our definition of psychoanalytic work is going to be. Some authors feel an understandable 'deep concern related to an obvious and increasing dilution of psychoanalysis' (Argentieri & Amati Mahler 2003, p. 19). However, once we abide to certain basic principles (theoretical, such as the belief in the power of unconscious phantasies; technical, such as the importance of offering a consistent setting; and ethical, such as the obligation to respect confidentiality), I believe that any definition of our psychoanalytic work must allow for a modicum of flexibility.

Over the years, psychoanalysis has been characterised as that form of non-directive 'talking cure' that takes place with the patient lying on the couch (though some patients choose to be sitting face-to-face), for 50-minute-long sessions occurring five times a week (though some analysts also see patients less frequently, and for shorter sessions), accompanied by listening in a state of free-floating attention to the patient's free associations (though it is acknowledged that all sorts of modalities of communication also occur as a norm). Transference interpretations constitute the main interventions (though analysts also make different kinds of interventions all the time, such as reconstructions and asking indirect questions) with an initially open-ended contract as a condition (though some analysts also agree to see patients for only a limited period of time or number of sessions). *Et cetera.*

What constitutes 'true' analysis has to be seen in the context of a rapidly evolving environment, where new technologies, and the culture and values associated with them, cannot be ignored as they play such an important part not only in our practical daily lives and in our interpersonal relationships, but also in the structure and contents of our internal worlds. Psychoanalysis in its traditional form might soon become a curiosity from the past. But if we, the few remaining digital immigrants, collaborate with the natives in responding proactively to the electronic revolution, then our beloved impossible profession still has a good chance to thrive.

References

Argentieri, S. and Amati Mehler, J. (2003). Telephone 'analysis': 'Hello, who's speaking?' *Insight, 12*(1): 17–19.

Bassen, C. (2007). Telephone analysis. Panel report. *Journal of the American Psychoanalytic Association, 55*: 1033–1041.

Carlino, R. (2010). *Distance psychoanalysis*. London: Karnac.

Fornari-Spoto, G. (2011). *The Bulletin of the British Psychoanalytical Society, 47*: 7–11.

Freud, S. (1912). Recommendations to physicians practising psycho-analysis. *Standard Edition, 12*: 109–120.

Leffert, M. (2003). Analysis and psychotherapy by telephone: twenty years of clinical experience. *Journal of the American Psychoanalytic Association, 51*: 101–130.

Prensky, M. (2001). Digital natives, digital immigrants. *On the Horizon*, 9(5): 1–6.

Sabbadini, A. (1989). Boundaries of timelessness. Some thoughts about the temporal dimension of the psychoanalytic space. *International Journal of Psychoanalysis*, 70(2): 305–313.

Scharff, J. (2010). Telephone analysis. Panel report. *International Journal of Psychoanalysis*, *91*: 989–992.

Vinocur Fischbein, S. (2010). Psychoanalysis and virtual reality. Panel report. *International Journal of Psychoanalysis*, *91*: 985–988.

Yamin Habib, L. (2003). Physical presence – a sine qua non of analysis? *Insight, 12*(1): 25–27.

Zalusky, S. (2003). Dialogue: Telephone analysis. *Insight, 12*(1): 13–16.

Chapter 2

Cyberpassion

E-rotic transference and the internet

Glen Gabbard

While psychoanalysis has generally been regarded as "the talking cure," written communication from patient to analyst commonly appears within the analytic setting. In our electronic age, e-mail communications from patient to analyst have become commonplace. This paper describes a case of erotic transference conveyed primarily through e-mail messages, and discusses their multiple meanings as an enactment. The unique features of e-mail communication are explored and contrasted with verbal discourse in the analytic dyad.

The playwright Sam Shepard recently made the following observation: "The struggle with the land is finished ... Now the frontier is the computer, so it has become an internal thing. Computers cause protracted dreaming about what might be, and the frontier everyone is seeking is now in the imagination" (Weber 2000, p. 10).

California may still be the epicenter of the frontier, but the Gold Rush now takes place in virtual space. The lore from Silicon Valley is that the region produces 60 freshly minted millionaires a day. Virtual communities are springing up in this new nevernever land, leading to new definitions of intimacy. The discourse on the Internet between two individuals sitting at computers in distant locations is not exactly *in* the world, but it is not exactly *outside* the world either. Indeed, the undefined boundaries of cyberspace offer new possibilities.

It was only a matter of time until psychotherapeutic treatments went online. A small but growing literature has developed on such topics as *Internet regression* and *transference on the Internet* (Childress 1998; Laszlo, Esterman, & Zabko 1999; Polauf 1998; Suler 1998). The absence of information about the person on the other end of the e-mail communication and the lack of visual cues facilitate the attribution of various qualities to the other person. Anger, narcissistic wounds, and feelings of rejection are commonplace in e-mail communications.

Parallel with the growth of advice giving and psychotherapy on the Internet has been the widely publicized phenomenon of cybersex, and even cybersex addiction (Toomey & Rothenberg 2000). One-third of adult Internet visits are to sexually oriented chat rooms, websites, and news groups (Brody 2000). Cloaked in anonymity, total strangers can express their unbridled sexual fantasies to each other with a candor that would be unthinkable in the physical presence of another person. The immediacy of online communication and the disinhibiting effect of talking online (Grohol 1998), two characteristics frequently associated with the Internet, undoubtedly contribute to the popularity of this mode of communication. We now hear of men and women who fall passionately in love with "cyber pen pals" whom they have never seen.

The literature has addressed the effects of other media (diaries and letters, telephone calls) as forms of enactment in psychoanalytic treatment. However, up to this time, there has been a paucity of literature attempting to describe the effects of new developments on the Internet regarding analytic treatment. Nevertheless, many analysts have been confronted with situations in which patients have communicated through e-mail, creating the need for analysts to develop creative solutions of their own. In this communication, I address two parallel developments in this new era of cyberspace in which most of us find ourselves living: the use of e-mail in clinical settings, and the facilitation of sexual expression made possible by communication through cyberspace.

While I did not seek out this new ground for exploration, I nevertheless had to confront such a variation on the expression of erotic transference in the course of my clinical work. My intent is not to propose a definitive technical approach to this phenomenon, but only to share my struggles with unfamiliar territory and to make a contribution to what is bound to be an ongoing dialog on this subject.

Clinical illustration

Rachel was an academic at a nearby university who came to analysis in her mid-thirties. She had been in analysis for a little over a year when she began to develop the glimmerings of erotic transference. She told me of her wish to be special and unique among all my patients. With considerable inhibition and halting speech, she wanted to know if I loved her. She found it extremely difficult to elaborate on her feelings toward me, and often ridiculed the analytic mode of talking instead of acting. She insisted that she would be able to talk to me more openly if we were sexually involved. She said that if I were to make love to her, she would then have solid evidence that I cared about her.

Rachel came to one session and announced, "I think the only reason you won't go to bed with me is that you don't like me and don't want me sexually. I can't talk about what I want from you, so I brought a song lyric to read to you." She then read the following:

> The sparrows chirp and the chipmunks chatter
> And we go on as mad as a hatter
> And nothing at all gets said.

> Talk to me in bed
> Where it matters.

She went on to compare her love for me to a nun's love for Christ, and expressed exasperation that nothing was going to develop from this.

The day after she read the song lyric to me, I arrived at my office and read my e-mail, as I always do. I was surprised to find the following message from her:

> You have undoubtedly noticed that I clam up at times, and you probably attribute it to embarrassment. Actually, while I am only mildly reluctant to share personal feelings with you, I am utterly unable to talk about them. I seem to have a real taboo on speech. It helps if you put words in my mouth. Once the topic is on the table, I can usually elaborate, to some degree.

When she arrived for her session that day, Rachel asked if I had seen the e-mail message, and I replied that indeed I had. She asked if I could help her by putting words to some of her sexual fantasies about me. I told her that I thought I could be of more help if she could elaborate on the difficulties she experienced in trying to talk about her fantasies. She said she was terrifically "turned on" in our last session, and felt that a sadomasochistic interaction was occurring because of my frustration of her erotic wishes: "You're encouraging me to be frustrated, and it seems odd to talk about it, but not to act on the feelings."

Rachel was a highly intelligent and classically educated woman. She had read widely about psychoanalysis. She commented that she fully understood the principle of transference, and went on to add: "I don't really think it has to be incestuous if you and I become sexually involved. You're not my father. If we had sex, you would be *you*—not a figure contaminated by transference. I just can't talk about sex; I do not have the vocabulary for it. I've never been able to use words for sex organs or intercourse, even with C [her current lover, with whom she lived] or with previous lovers."

I noted that it *did* seem that Rachel had a much stronger taboo about saying things than about writing them in e-mail communications. I wondered if she had any thoughts about this speech taboo.

Rachel then said that her mother used to refer to certain things as "unspeakable," and she specifically did not want to hear about what Rachel had done. One of her favorite comments was, "Ask me no questions, and I'll tell you no lies." Rachel went on, "Sometimes, in the evening, my mother would sit down at the piano and play this song that had the words 'We don't talk about that.' In our house, we didn't talk about lots of things." Rachel paused, and after a minute or two, I asked, "What things didn't you talk about?"

Rachel hesitated before saying, "There's something I haven't really told you about. When I was three or four, I slept in my brother's bed, off and on for about two years. He would have been about seven or eight when this started. He was really my first love. He would seduce me wordlessly, and I would silently go along with him. But I did enjoy it. At some level, I knew it was wrong, but it seemed natural at another level. It provided me with something that I desperately need from you now. My mother was emotionally sadistic with me; I was repeatedly buoyed up and dashed down by her fickleness, over which I had no control. To some extent, I repeat this now with you. Without your doing anything but analyzing, I go through cycles of feeling loved and then rejected."

I pointed out to her that she *was* able to talk about very intense feelings, and even about the incestuous behavior with her brother, and I wondered why she had felt the need to send an e-mail to me, rather than telling me her feelings in person. She responded, "I told you before—I cannot talk about sex. I had planned to overcome my reluctance in using explicitly sexual language in my e-mail message, but I couldn't make myself do it. The words didn't sound like me."

Rachel equated her inhibition about sexual talk with secret keeping, noting that the sexual relationship with her brother was something that was kept secret from her mother. At times, she felt it was the only thing that her mother did not know about her. In a subsequent e-mail to me, Rachel noted that the incestuous relationship:

> gave me an identity separate from her—an act of rebellion that defined who I am. It's a new experience to not act on the feelings I have toward you. I'd rather have you on the analytic couch, making love to me. I can show you how I feel, but it's much harder to tell you. I really long to submit to you. I love to call you "Dr. Gabbard" because it elevates you above me, which is a turn-on.

At the next session after this message was sent, Rachel asked me if I had liked its content. She then added provocatively, "Remember—I'm ready to submit any time." I replied, "But submitting to me carries with it the same concern that you had with your mother—namely, that you will lose your separate identity and disappear."

Rachel answered, "I don't have a sense of who I am; I don't have a sense of self. With my mother, I always felt I'd already lost myself. I couldn't possibly feel separate from her. I think of analysis differently, almost as an opportunity to get rid of myself and merge with you, since I'm tired of being me. Sex with you would accomplish that. It would be secret; no one would know but us."

I said, "Much like your relationship with your brother."

In the ensuing months following this exchange, I regularly received e-mail messages from Rachel in between her sessions. Much of the content involved her passionate sexual desire toward me and her inability to talk about this directly in the sessions. Here is an example:

> You may be wondering if I'm still going around lovestruck and wet all the time. Sure. I'm wanting you terrifically, and I spent most of today thinking about you and masturbating. I had the house to myself as C was on a business trip, so I was able to walk around nude. It was very stimulating, and I wished you were there. I had planned in this message to try to overcome my reluctance in using sexually explicit language, but it didn't sound like me. I want you to talk dirty to me. I know you're going away at the end of next week, and I'd like to make love with you before you go. It drives me crazy that it's just talk.

As implied by this last message, the intensity of the erotic feelings seemed to increase prior to my absences, and especially during my absences. Here is one of the messages that was sent while I was out of the country at a meeting:

> You've only been away for one and a half days, and I already miss you terribly. It feels like I'm in love. When I'm driving to your office, I start thinking about you and expecting sex. My body has certain sensations. There is a tingly sensation on the skin of my breasts, stomach, and thighs, and an empty feeling inside my lower abdomen and mouth. It seems to be specific to you; I haven't noticed it happening in regard to anyone else.
>
> After considering the various possibilities in your office, I've decided that the best spot for lovemaking would be on the Oriental rug. We would have plenty of room to move around and engage in foreplay. On second thought, foreplay would be like teasing to me in this state of mind. Afterplay would be fun, though.
>
> I bought one of your books, and I envy the male patient in your book who could speak so freely about sex. It seems that I have a stronger taboo about saying things than doing them. I would love to perform fellatio on you (for my own pleasure, not just yours), but I couldn't come near to describing the act. One of my former lovers noticed my inarticulateness and tutored me in this area. He'd ask me if I wanted certain sexual things, and he would tell me to parrot back his words. I never could say those words for sexual acts independently, but it was still a terrific turn-on for me. Am I allowed to get turned on in sessions?

One of the obvious functions of these e-mail communications was to maintain a connection in fantasy with me during my absences, as well as between sessions. When Rachel sent me a message, it created for her a sense of being present in my mind. As we analyzed the meaning of her e-mail correspondence, she observed that "email is a direct line to you—*always*—wherever you are. I don't have to risk interrupting you at home with your wife and kids, as I would on the phone. I always felt overheard by my mom as a kid when I spoke to friends over the phone. But e-mail seems more private."

Bringing cyberspace communication into the analytic space

From my perspective, these messages presented a dilemma. I felt that the analysis of this extra-analytic communication was essential, and the patient's thoughts and fantasies could not remain *outside* the analytic process. On the other hand, Rachel felt incapable of putting these thoughts into words in our sessions. I did not want to start an adjunctive e-mail analysis by dealing with this material via Internet correspondence; hence, I told the patient that the material she sent me in e-mails should be brought into the analysis so that we could discuss it. A compromise was worked out: she would print her messages and bring them to me as hard copies. I would read what she wrote, and together we would analyze the material.

This approach led to highly productive explorations of the various meanings of words versus actions, writing versus speaking, and the use of the e-mail medium itself. For example, writing had the connotation to Rachel of being more permanent and less likely to be ignored. She observed, "One thing I like about e-mail is that you *get* every word I say, unlike verbal communication, where you don't really take in everything I speak. That's especially important in a love letter."

Rachel was able to express her concern that if she voiced her sexual feelings in my presence, I might violate sexual boundaries with her, and then she would be responsible for ruining my career. I pointed out to her that responsibility for maintaining boundaries resides with the analyst rather than with the patient. She responded that in childhood, she had always been responsible for her mother's emotions because her mother was unstable. She could endure pain better than her mother could, being the stronger of the two.

Rachel also stressed that e-mail communication relieved her of responsibility in another sense. In one session, she reflected on the difference between typing an e-mail to me and verbalizing her passion in the session, saying of the former: "It's out there, and it's already in the past. Therefore, I don't have to be responsible for it."

We also came to understand how e-mail functioned as a self-preservative barrier to intimacy. Rachel was able to draw an analogy between her reluctance to lose herself to me in sexual talk and her fear of surrendering to orgasm. She commented that she preserved a sense of self by using e-mail and avoiding frankly erotic dialog with me. She rarely had orgasms, and she had frequently said that she wished to avoid orgasm because it carried with it a threat of losing the self. In one session, she commented, "I hated the loss of control when I first had an orgasm. In masturbation, there's much less of a threat of losing a sense of who I am. I know it's hard for men to understand why a woman would not want to have an orgasm. But it's hard for me to expose myself to that extent; I value my privacy. One of the reasons I have such a hard time free associating in analysis is that it feels like I'd be giving up all my privacy." Hence, from the patient's perspective, e-mail preserved a sense of privacy and bypassed the free-association process, which she felt would be a catastrophic capitulation in which she would lose all control and even a solid sense of who she was.

Throughout the analysis of her inhibition about talking, Rachel continued to push for action. She commented that she sexualized our relationship because she could not feel close unless we had sex, noting that a similar feeling had been involved during her incestuous relationship with her brother. She recalled that it was the only way of being close with him in a family in which she felt close to no one. If I had sex with her, she would know that I cared. She also knew that I would always remember her because she would be an anomaly in my practice. I pointed out to her that in a similar way, her use of e-mail to communicate with me might carry with it a powerful fantasy of being unique, special, and perhaps unforgettable.

It was apparent to both Rachel and me that even though her sexual wishes were not consummated in the analysis, to some extent, she was able to introduce action through the Internet. Typing e-mails to me was unequivocally an *act*. My reading the e-mails aloud to her was also an enactment of a sexualized relationship. In her fantasies, she loved to think of me as a dominant figure who would force her to submit. In my insistence that the e-mail letters should not remain outside of the process, we were enacting a dominance–submission paradigm that at some level was highly gratifying to her. In one session, she commented, "I'm sure you don't use the caveman approach I like when making love, but at least when you make me go through these messages, I can feel like you're a caveman forcing this stuff on me."

While her observation was certainly valid, I believed that my decision had been the enactment of choice in a smorgasbord of problematic options. If I did not insist on bringing the messages into the analytic discourse, I would be enacting a secretive, exclusive relationship with Rachel that re-created the incestuous bond with her brother. I also came to recognize that she had an intense feeling of shame associated with her attempts to talk about love and sexual desire in person with me. In one of her e-mails, she recollected her experience with her mother:

> My tender feelings were always ridiculed [by her] as sentimental and foolish, so now I feel bad about my feelings that I am "in love" with you. I also feel foolish and subject to ridicule from you. That is worse to me than a Scarlet Letter type of ostracism.

Communicating her feelings through the Internet moderated Rachel's shame and protected her from what she felt was inevitable humiliation by me.

Countertransference in cyberspace

While I noted in my introductory comments that there is a growing literature on transference in cybercommunication, almost nothing has been written about countertransference in that sphere. My receipt of sexually charged e-mails from Rachel felt illicit in some way. There was a part of me that felt I needed to close my door while I read her messages. What would a colleague think who dropped in unexpectedly and saw what I was reading? At times, I felt I was reading pornographic communications, and I would be aware of a sense of embarrassment. I recalled news stories of corporate employees who had been fired for accessing pornographic sites during work hours. I would feel a pressing need to delete her e-mails from my computer system as soon as possible, in order to avoid discovery, partly in the name of preserving the patient's confidentiality, but partly to deal with my own sense of shame at deriving a special form of secret excitement from reading them.

I recognized a part of me that wanted to collude with Rachel in a subtle subversion of the analytic task staged in cyberspace, where nobody would ever know. Steiner (2000) suggested that in most analysts, hate for analysis coexists with love. The analytic enterprise demands a discipline and restraint that is highly frustrating. Each of us has a host of competing agendas when we sit behind the couch, and I found myself struggling with my own conflicting needs in the analysis with Rachel.

Over time, I noticed—to my surprise—that reading the letters out loud with the patient tended to dissipate my sexual excitement. Love letters are meant to be read in private, and the act of bringing them into the light of day and sharing them openly somehow diffuses the erotic element.

When Rachel finally began to put her sexual longings into words in our sessions, her secret e-mail messages—which were to some degree an unmentalized enactment akin to incest with her brother—were transformed into a relationship that could be reflected upon. In using these spoken words, she felt exposed and vulnerable. She gradually came to see, however, that I was not invested in shaming her, and she became more collaborative. The e-mail communications became less frequent over time and ultimately subsided, as though they had performed an important function in one phase of the analysis, but were no longer necessary.

Discussion

Psychoanalysis has long been referred to as "the talking cure," and there can be little doubt that Freud privileged verbal expression. Nevertheless, we must keep in mind that Freud's self-analysis took place largely in an epistolary relationship with Fliess (Perez 1992). Moreover, in Freud's analysis of Marie Bonaparte, the patient brought in her youthful notebooks and went over her writings with Freud during the hours (de Bissy 1990). I maintain that it would be a serious mistake to view the written communication of patients as merely a form of resistance or acting out.

Early in my career as an analytic candidate, one of my supervisors told me the story of a woman he had treated who brought a shoe box full of letters to the first session. She had wanted him to read the letters with her, and he had declined, suggesting that she instead tell him about their contents. The patient left and never returned. Some years later, he learned that she had committed suicide. He said that he had always wondered if going over the letters with her might have made a difference.

In the case of Rachel, there was an insistence on her part that my willingness to read her e-mails and incorporate them into the process made a huge difference to her. Some time after she stopped sending them to me, she reflected back on what had transpired:

> I would have felt shamed or slapped on the wrist if you had rejected my e-mails. I was expressing an aspect of me that I couldn't articulate verbally. If you had slammed the door shut on that hidden part of me, you would have been just like my mother. The message would have been that you were more interested in having me meet your requirements than in getting to know who I was. I would have felt like I'd failed as a patient.

Winnicott (1960) noted that infants whose initiatives are consistently thwarted by parents who cannot receive or validate them will find an alternative pathway to connect with their parents. This strategy usually involves the development of a false self whom the parents recognize and appreciate. The true self becomes shrouded in shame, however, and some degree of authenticity is lost.

Rachel's sexual writing can be viewed as a developmental step that needed to be taken prior to expression of her passion in speech. Her sexualized e-mail messages were repeating in action something that could not be verbalized. Her incestuous involvement with her brother was a wordless, secret, and forbidden relationship that also served the function of maintaining a sense of defiance of and separateness from her mother. To a large extent, a feeling of aliveness emanated from this relationship to fight off psychological deadness, as well as engulfment by her mother's scrutiny and control. The incestuous behavior with her brother interfered with the developmentally appropriate frustration of desire that produces a capacity to delay. In her desperation to feel loved and validated, she turned to her brother, where she was prematurely overstimulated. My absences re-evoked the need to sexualize as a way to fend off feelings of deadness, disconnection, and loss (Gabbard 1996).

Rachel bypassed a developmental step in which such feelings could be processed and metabolized with fantasies and with words.

Bollas (1997) made the following observation:

> Part of the talking cure is in the innumerable precise and discrete emphases of the telling that "put" or "bring" the latent contents into discourse. The effect of this transportation gives new body to the analysand's speech, as it assists the patient in bringing the force of instincts into words adequate to bear and transform them, as well as bringing the force of the instinct into that poetics of telling that is in itself a derivative of sexual life.
>
> (p. 366)

In the analytic setting, the use of words to talk about erotic longings has a potentially transformative power. In the case of Rachel, however, that transformation was resisted with formidable resolve.

While we generally think of the verbalization of wishes and affects as having the potential to tame powerful feelings, in Rachel's case, the opposite was true. She was deeply conflicted about verbalization of sexual desire. On one hand, she longed to share her feelings with me, but on the other, she feared that giving words to her desire would result in unbridled discharge of her impulses that would either destroy my career or lead to her humiliation. For her, sexual longing was embodied more in the voice than in the written word, making Internet communication relatively safer.

In a discussion of the use of writing by adolescents, Litowitz and Gundlach (1987) described an important developmental aspect of writing, as follows.

> As there is a lessening of affect through mediation from experience to speech, there is a further weakening of affect in writing. Writing can therefore serve to tame and control emotions that threaten to overwhelm the subject. Writing, serving as a substitute action, can inhibit another action.
>
> (p. 86)

For Rachel, the medium of cyberspace was less affectively charged, and thus less likely to precipitate a sense of grief at having to give up the treasured but secret internal object relationship associated with incestuous sexuality.

Rachel's difficulty in using words to symbolize the transference was also reflected in her perception of the frequent collapse of the analytic "play space." The loss of the "as-if" nature of the transference was particularly striking in her insistence that if we made love, I would not be her father or her brother—I would simply be myself, "uncontaminated by transference."

Other analysts have commented on the role that writing may play in analysis. Figueiredo (1998) noted that spoken language has more immediacy than written language, where a certain amount of distance is possible. Putti (1998) shared my view that the analyst must bring written messages into the analysis for discussion. While she noted that motives for writing can include fear of the analyst's reaction and fear of the patient's own emotionality, she also stressed that trust in the analyst may be increased when the communications are read through together. Bertrand (1998) emphasized that a written narrative is a solitary act that involves no interactional risks. But how solitary is writing? Litowitz and Gundlach (1987) noted that the privacy of writing creates distance and the *appearance* of solitude, but that there is always an imaginary audience; hence, writing is always social and dialogic. They also suggested that writing differs from speech in that it leaves a visual trace that endures over time and space, while also allowing greater control over the consequences of the expression.

For Rachel, the physical absence of the analyst while she typed e-mail messages created a sense of space in which to find herself, apart from the analyst's immediate influence. She commented at one point, "When you say something in here, I have to pull back and decide if I really agree with what you're attributing to me, or if I am simply thinking it because *you* thought it. I used to think Mom was omniscient and could make me think what she thought. E-mail helps me think my *own* thoughts." Freedom of thought is a major goal of analytic work (Symington 1990), and communication via e-mail helped Rachel to achieve that goal.

Unique aspects of e-mail communication

While e-mail writing has much in common with other forms of writing in analysis, it also has some unique properties. Lear (2000) pointed out that the physical use of the fingers is closely related to the discharge of impulses. He noted that many people regret having hit the "send" button on their computers too soon, wishing that they had delayed the impulse with greater thought and anticipation of consequences. Indeed, the Internet disinhibits one's defense mechanisms and allows for greater disclosure than in ordinary discourse (Uecker 1997). As demonstrated by Rachel's case, e-mail communication allows one to overcome shame and other inhibiting factors that prevent direct expression of embarrassing feelings in person.

Furthermore, the use of passwords and online identities allows for the illusion of a secret, forbidden relationship with an e-mail pen pal. Rachel told me in one of her e-mails not to hit the "reply" button if I responded, because her lover might see what she had written. She very much conveyed the sense of hiding an affair. Of course, such privacy is only illusory because the confidentiality of e-mails is roughly equivalent to the confidentiality of a postcard; after an e-mail is sent, it does not disappear, but is traceable and identifiable. After the message is read, a copy usually remains behind on the Internet service provider's computer or on the online service's computer (Labruzza 1997).

Even deleted messages can be retrieved. Finally, messages are frequently sent to the wrong person, with the potential to cause great embarrassment.

These considerations raise profound concerns about the trend toward conducting psychotherapy over the Internet. Case law is still evolving in this area, but in Rachel's case, I had serious reservations about sending any kind of significant communication via e-mail because of the potential for a breach of confidentiality. I generally limited my replies to her to an acknowledgment that I had received the message.

The use of a screen persona reflects another unique phenomenon associated with cybercommunication: permission to develop a playful expansion of the self. In the case of Rachel, the screen persona was her, but at the same time, not her. As Turkle (1997) put it, "You can have a sense of self without being one self" (p. 258). Turkle (1984) reinterpreted the story of Narcissus by noting that the mythological subject did not really fall in love with himself—he fell in love with an image that appeared to him to be someone else. Similarly, while looking into the computer screen, we can play with the idea of becoming someone other than who we are. Indeed, we may be searching for ourselves as we look into the computer screen and try on different identities to communicate with others. Virtual space has a lot in common with transitional space, in the sense that it is not truly an internal realm, but lies somewhere between external reality and our internal world. When we sit at a computer, we are both real and not real. Using e-mail, Rachel was able to try on a new version of herself that included the ability to directly express passionate sexual desire, an ability that she ultimately integrated and made a part of herself.

A similar paradox exists around the nature of the object to whom one is writing. The person sending an e-mail message is alone, but not alone. The apparent privacy allows for freer expression, but the awareness of the other receiving the e-mail allows for passionate attachment and highly emotional expressiveness. The Internet has led to new definitions of privacy as well as of intimacy.

Rachel's cybercommunication expanded the boundary of the analytic experience. As I struggled with matters of confidentiality, sexual excitement, and the feeling that I was colluding in some form of secret cybersex, I was aware of my own anxieties about expanding and redefining the boundaries of analysis. Was I transgressing a boundary by incorporating e-mail communication into analysis, or was I breaking new ground on the analytic frontier in a constructive and creative way?

Conclusion

The use of e-mail communication in the course of an analysis can have multiple meanings, as can any other form of enactment. In the case of Rachel, it re-created a forbidden relationship that had allowed her to survive a childhood dominated by a stifling and intrusive mother. It also provided a medium in which to express burning passion that could not be put into words. It simultaneously provided a sense of omnipotent control over her analyst, since in her fantasy, it would keep me from acting on her provocations while also providing an attenuated sadomasochistic interaction—one in which I "forced" her to analyze what she had written. E-mail communication also maintained a connection between us during my absences, thus serving to deny our separateness. Paradoxically, it created a separate space for Rachel to define herself apart from me. The typing of e-mail messages created a transitional space for her in which she could play with new versions of herself.

Turkle (1984, 1997) compared the cultural impact of the computer to that of psychoanalysis. Freud offered new ways for people to think about themselves, which included helping them to deal with guilt about sexual aspects of the self. Turkle suggested that cybercommunication is expanding the self in new ways, since ultimately, it forces us to take a hard look at what it means to be human. If Sam Shepard (Weber 2000) is correct that the new frontier lies in the realm of the imagination, we psychoanalysts should be around for a good long time, since that territory is one of our favorite stomping grounds.

References

Bertrand, M. (1998). Valeurs et limites du narratif en psychanalyse. *Revue Français Psychanalyse*, *62*: 713–720.

Bollas, C. (1997). Wording and telling sexuality. *International Journal of Psycho-Analysis*, *78*: 363–367.

Brody, J. E. (2000). Cybersex gives birth to a psychological disorder. *New York Times*, May 16.

Childress, C. (1998). Potential risks and benefits of online psychotherapeutic interventions. Retrieved from http://www.ismho.org/issues/9801.htm.

de Bissy, G. (1990). La rememoration chez Marie Bonaparte et ses sinq cahiers. *Revue Français Psychanalyse, 54*: 1057–1071.

Figueiredo, L. C. (1998). A complexa nocao de "voz." *Revista Brasileria de Psicanalise*, *32*: 605–609.

Gabbard, G. O. (1996). *Love and hate in the analytic setting*. Northvale, NJ: Aronson.

Grohol, J. M. (1998). Future clinical directions: Professional development, pathology, and psychotherapy online. In J. Gackenbach (Ed.) *Psychology and the Internet: Intrapersonal, interpersonal, and transpersonal implications* (pp. 111–140). New York: Academic Press.

Labruzza, A. L. (1997). *The essential Internet: A Guide for psychotherapists and other mental health professionals*. Northvale, NJ: Aronson.

Laszlo, J. V., Esterman, G. & Zabko, S. (1999). Therapy over the Internet? Theory, research, and finances. *Cyber Psychology and Behavior*, *2*: 293–307.

Lear, J. (2000). Personal communication.

Litowitz, B. E. & Gundlach, R. A. (1987). When adolescents write: Semiotic and social dimensions of adolescents' personal writing. *Adolescent Psychiatry*, *14*: 82–111.

Perez, C. D. (1992). Soledades: Freud escritor de cartas. *Revista de Psicoanalisis*, *49*: 35–48.

Polauf, F. J. (1998). Psychotherapy on the Internet: Theory and technique. Available at http://www.nyreferrals.com/psychotherapy.

Putti, S. (1998). Comunicazioni scritte in analisi. *Giornale Storico di Psicologia Dinamica*, *22*: 149–157.

Steiner, J. (2000). Book review of A Mind of One's Own: A Kleinian View of Self and Object, by R. Caper. *Journal of the American Psychoanalytic Association.*, *48*: 637–643.

Suler, J. (1998). Mom, dad, computer: Transference reactions to computers. Retrieved from http://www.rider.edu/users/suler/psycyber/comptransf.html.

Symington, N. (1990). The possibility of human freedom and its transmission (with particular reference to the thought of Bion). *International Journal of Psycho-Analysis*, *71*: 95–106.

Toomey, K. E. & Rothenberg, R. B. (2000). Sex and cyberspace—virtual networks leading to high-risk sex. *Journal of the American Medical Association*, *284*: 485–487.

Turkle, S. (1984). *The second self: Computers and the human spirit*. New York: Simon & Schuster.

Turkle, S. (1997). *Life on the screen: Identity and the age of the Internet*. New York: Touchtone.

Uecker, E. Z. (1997). Psychodynamic considerations of online counseling. Retrieved from http://www.cmhc.com/perspective/article/arto1971.html.

Weber, B. (2000). An unusual case of role reversal. *New York Times*, February 27, p. 10.

Winnicott, D. W. (1960). *The maturational processes and the facilitating environment: Studies in the theory of emotional development*. London: Hogarth.

Chapter 3

Clinical issues in analyses over the telephone and the internet

Jill Savege Scharff

The use of technology in psychoanalysis

The development of a global economy with increased travel and instant worldwide communication has produced a social and personal transformation of the mind and its concept of the body in space. This governs the mind-set and lifestyle of analysands to which psychoanalysts must now adapt their treatment approach. So, psychoanalysis has to find ways of transcending the limits of distance to reach the analysand of the 21st century. Possible solutions are to diminish the frequency of sessions (more like psychotherapy), condense them into periods of availability (condensed analysis), or require travel by analyst or analysand (remote condensed shuttle analysis). Another solution is to maintain frequency through the use of communication by voice, using the telephone or the Internet, possibly including the use of a one-way or two-way camera. Harnessing technology to the analytic aim may be a creative adaptation to the modern world but it raises many questions concerning the viability of the frame, the emergence of resistance, the maintenance of the therapeutic alliance, the sensitivity of response to unconscious communication of affect and fantasy without non-verbal cues, and the development of analytic process (Scharff 2010).

Technology has been used in conducting psychoanalytic sessions for six decades but its acceptability was limited for years by available equipment, ethical concerns, and paucity of data about its effectiveness. There is no doubt that in-person sound is more comfortable to listen to, but the analyst can adapt to telephone communication for analytic sessions when necessary. In the 1950s the first report of the use of the telephone in psychoanalysis recommended the speaker phone as the closest approximation to in-person sound (Saul 1951). A cluster of reports appeared in the 1970s (Robertiello 1972–1973) and an edited book on the telephone in intensive psychotherapy at the turn of the century (Aronson 2000a). The telephone was used as needed for dealing with crises and reaching a reluctant or bed-ridden patient. It was seen as an extension of the transitional space (Aronson 2000b). It was used as a substitute for in-person analysis for patients who were phobic of in-person sessions.

It was used with patients who had to move so that they could maintain an established analytic relationship and prevent premature termination. Lindon (2000) reported in detail on the analysis of a single case with serious pathology in which he dealt with a transference filled with anger, disgust, contempt, paranoid fantasies, and fears of engulfment. In contrast, Leffert (2003) reported on nine analyses in which he found that telephone sessions were indistinguishable from in-person sessions, but he did not support his findings with detailed process. Even though he had shown the power of telephone analysis, Lindon (2000) thought it second-best. Benson, Rowntree, and Singer (2001) who saw its value and Zalusky (1998) who is an advocate for the appropriate use of the telephone in psychoanalysis nevertheless regarded it as a therapeutic compromise. Disagreeing with such a modest assessment, Sachs (2003) cautioned that this view of telephone analysis may "overemphasize being cautious in its use and totally diminish its value" (p. 29). Most writers recommend a trial of telephone sessions before agreeing to switch from in-person sessions, with periodic return to in-person sessions on a flexible schedule.

In 2003, the use of a telephone headset attachment was being recommended as being "operationally transparent" and offering a superior sense of connection (Leffert 2003, p. 117). By 2011, the headset was commonly in use by analyst and analysand, but connected not only to the telephone landlines but also to the Internet, using Voice Over Internet Protocol (VOIP)[1]. The telephone distorts the inflection of the voice, and critics fear that this will interfere with the reception of the communication (Argentieri & Mehler 2003). VOIP has the advantage that it is a secure method of communication that provides high fidelity stereo sound by using more megahertz than telephone lines, and this means that the voice on VOIP is startlingly vivid. When it enters the headset, the voice of the analysand is delivered inside the analyst's mind in a more total way than in the room where there is more space between them and visual input as well. Varela (personal communication 2007) holds that the analyst's voice coming straight through the headset into the analysand's ear fosters a sense of connection that supports the containment offered by the analytic process.

Furthermore, VOIP now offers analyst and analysand the choice of visual transmission by using a web camera so that analysand and analyst can see each other at the beginning and end of the session and the analyst can look at the analysand's body movements as the web camera is trained on the analysand's couch. Some analysts, even those in the United States with analysands as far away as in China, find that this degree of physical communication approximates closely to that of the in-person analytic session (Snyder 2011). Nevertheless there is a slight delay, the image is fuzzier than in person, and accompanying odors are not conveyed. Other analysts find the telephone more evocative of the in-person session in which looking and seeing are less important than following and responding to verbal associations with unconscious fantasies and communicable thoughts.

Technical difficulties occur in using the telephone or the Internet. Whichever method is chosen, analyst and analysand may experience upsetting moments of dropped connection or extraneous noises on the telephone line and in the broadband connection supporting VOIP. These problems are the technical equivalent of an empathic failure, but even technical failure can bring the transference into focus, as the following example shows.

Clinical process: a technical problem

Mr. M, an adult male analysand with trauma-related depression, began analysis in person and moved to telephone analysis while still in the early phase of treatment, because his company sent him to work in an area with no local analyst. He attended four times a week by telephone, and returned in person for a week three times a year. His communication in person and on the phone at this stage of treatment was characterized by quiet speech, many pauses, long silences, and only a few dreams.

Mr. M grew up in an industrial region known for its toxic air, which left him sickly. His father worked long hours at the factory and his mother took care of him on her own, her own family being across in Canada. As a child, he felt a nuisance to his mother. Being a quiet boy instead of a lively girl as his mother would have preferred, he felt that she did not love him. His life-threatening failure to thrive, accompanied by recurrent infections, required frequent hospitalizations, which must have exhausted her. One time when he had pneumonia, she left him in hospital where he was isolated in an oxygen tent and saw only nurses and doctors. When he tried to call out for her (which was hard because he could not breathe well on that occasion) he felt chastised by the nurses.

A telephone line cut-off happened early in his treatment. After some minutes of telling his analyst hesitantly what was on his mind, Mr. M fell silent. Hearing nothing from him, the analyst began to interpret the persistent use of silence as a resistance, as a denial of the need of the telephone and for words as the vehicle for the treatment, and as a way of testing her capacity to endure non-connection. Unbeknown to her, the analysand was speaking but the analyst could not hear him because her headset failed. He was puzzled by her ever more frantic attempts to interpret his non-response as his way of exerting silent control, making the telephone analysis impossible. After they discovered the problem and reconnected, the analyst learned that Mr. M had actually been speaking, and had been experiencing irritation in her voice as if she were not satisfied with what he was saying and not responding to him. The analyst was thinking of this as a vivid, concrete example of her "not getting it," not being able to tune in to him, an empathic failure. Feeling embarrassed, she apologized and said, "I must have sounded like a crazy person." This had resonance for him since, unbeknown to her, he indeed worried about making her crazy. However, mainly he felt that he was in trouble for not talking. He felt as he had felt in childhood when his "too quiet" way of being irritated his mother and drove her crazy. He had the sense that talking was pointless, since it seemed to make no impact even though he was desperately trying to communicate. So, these two sessions of telephone analysis brought into focus a transference view of himself as an unsatisfactory child, evoked a countertransference in identification with his irritated mother; and analysis of this transference–countertransference relieved its impact on the treatment alliance.

The development of analytic thinking about teleanalysis

The younger generation of analysands and analysts grew up conducting intimate communication on the phone, emailing and texting, and to them it is quite natural to call in to a business meeting, job interview, or psychoanalytic session from another location. They live on their cellphones and laptops, and when they travel for work, they cannot maintain the desired level of analytic frequency. Technology is driving their choices, and their lifestyle is driving their need for technology, including the need for technology-assisted psychoanalysis to maintain the optimum frequency of analytic sessions for in-depth analytic work. To comprehend their reality, some psychoanalysts are developing a sophisticated psychoanalytic understanding of the changing dimensions of time and space in the 21st century (Aryan et al. 2009; Aryan & Carlino 2010). They are exploring technology's effects on the social unconscious and on the individual mind, whether analyzed in person or on the phone. They are balancing the provision of an appropriate analytic stance and an appropriate response to the impact of sociocultural change on the patient, and on the analyst's identity and the nature of his practice (Rodriguez de la Sierra 2003).

Like traditional analysis in person, teleanalysis values the standard psychoanalytic tenets. Hanly (2007) found in his experience of telephone analysis that responsive holding, witnessing, and interpretive functions can be sustained, free association occurs, and the expression of paternal and maternal transferences are not compromised. Aryan (Aryan et al. 2009), Carlino (2011), and Lutenberg (2011a and b) agree that teleanalysis is similar to traditional analysis in using the analyst's suspended attention to free association, working with the unconscious and its derivatives and repressed childhood sexuality, and in analyzing dreams and transference. Mirkin (2011) thought that phone analysis provided a "relative protection from impulsive actions" and thereby "allowed intense affects to be expressed, tolerated and reflected upon" and "helped an exploration of defenses unfold" (p. 669). Even though the body is absent, the telephone session is effective because it echoes the "silent-but-holding environment presence of the mother" (Leffert 2003, p.10). Just as traditional psychoanalysis can be extended to treat analysands with pathology that is not classically neurotic, teleanalysis can be effective in perversion and psychosis in some cases. Symington, whose analysand had to travel after years of in-person psychoanalysis, found that the dislocation of being away from home and having to connect to him on the telephone revealed a transference delusion previously not brought out in the consulting room (Anderson et al. 2009). Richards (2003), who has had experience of telephone analysis and its supervision intermittently for years, reported on an analysis in which a sexual perversion, hidden in person, emerged only when encouraged to have telephone sessions with the analyst. Then it came to light that the patient had been having a covert form of telephone sex with her mother for years, unaware that her shuddering release was orgasmic.

Although analysis by telephone or VOIP has its proponents, it remains controversial, and like any proposed innovation, it has stirred lively debate. Conceding that the telephone might occasionally be a useful therapeutic tool, Argentieri and Mehler (2003) nevertheless concluded that it is not compatible with a psychoanalytic process and is traumatic for both analyst and patient. Their concern is that the offer of telephone sessions denies separation and loss, and at the same time creates loss in depriving the patient of the bodily presence of the analyst and therefore of good holding containment. Yamin Habib (2003) found that the stance of the telephone analyst is not properly authentic, neutral, and impartial: instead it is indulgent and paternalistic, privileging action and the exchange of information rather than providing a lived experience. Brainsky (2003) described the analytic relationship on the telephone as "an unusually spectral relationship" resulting from persecutory condensations of tone, timbre, and word that render the analyst's voice as a part-object (p. 23). He believed that telephone analysis is more likely than traditional analysis to result in idealized transference and to fail in the task of containing projective identifications.

Therapeutic regression occurs in analysis by telephone and on the Internet as it does in traditional analysis. However it must be admitted that this is more anxiety-provoking for the analyst, who may experience increased anxiety about doing harm and being censured. As Chodorow says of telephone analysis, "Regression can be really palpable, and sometimes, to me, scary … something you feel you can control more in the room" (2004, p. 4). More than anything, this anxious and guilty sensation translates into the commonly held view (despite a lack of research data) that in-person sessions are better.

Teleanalysis is not the same as analysis with the analysand in the consulting room, and yet it is more alike than different beyond surface characteristics. Leffert (2003) pointed out that "the telephone, like the couch, alters the dimensions of the non-verbal environment: it de-emphasizes or eliminates some of them while emphasizing others" (p.124). Communication occurs through sound, not sight, an echo of the earliest days of life when communication between mother and baby was perhaps through the whish of blood in the umbilical cord (Benaim 2009, personal communication). The telephone is like the couch in limiting visual cues and freeing the analyst's attention from the demands of gaze interaction (Richards 2003). The analyst listens with the third ear to the underlying theme, like the analyst sitting out of sight behind the analysand, listening better with eyes shut (Hanly 2007). As Freud put it, the analyst "must turn his own unconscious like a receptive organ towards the transmitting unconscious of the patient" (1912, p. 115), and "must adjust himself to the patient as a telephone receiver is adjusted to the transmitting microphone" (Freud 1912, pp. 115–116; Bollas 2009, personal communication). Zalusky (2000) linked the experience of telephone analysis unbounded by personal presence to "the timelessness of the unconscious" (p. 38). Each participant creates and sustains a mental representation of the other in fantasy, and analytic process develops in this new way as it does in traditional analysis (Zalusky 2003b).

Adaptation of frame, resistance and technique in teleanalysis

In teleanalysis, as in traditional analysis, the analyst respects the frame of the treatment and secures a circumscribed, reliable setting with regular frequency of sessions and time boundaries to each session, and an agreed routine for periods of in-person sessions. However, in teleanalysis, with the analyst and analysand in two different locations, there may be a considerable difference in the space, hour, and season of the setting for each of them (Aryan et al. 2009). Unlike traditional analysis in which the analyst provides and controls the setting, in analysis using the telephone or the Internet, the analyst and analysand think together about how to secure the frame, but analysands alone are responsible for the external arrangements; for securing the confidentiality of the at-home or in-office setting in which analysis occurs, for providing their own tissues, and if they choose to use a web camera, they are responsible for placing the couch suitably in relation to the camera. How they fulfill this responsibility is an expression of their endopsychic structure and their resistance, which can then be analyzed as usual. Chodorow (2004) reported that the analysand's creation of a physical surround – the room, the couch, the furniture, the light, the weather, the presence of pets, food, and drink – made her more aware of the analysand's sense of physical space (and of her own sense of her surroundings), than in in-person sessions where aspects of the shared space are taken for granted. Aspects of the analysand's location are evocative objects that become vehicles for understanding the psychological space that they reflect or protect against.

It has been said that in adapting the frame, teleanalysis accommodates to resistance instead of analyzing it, but the analyst analyzes both the need for the phone and the reluctance to use it when indicated. The request for telephone sessions may be a neurotic need, an enactment, an ego adaptation, or a mixture of defense and adaptation. Some analysands resist using the phone to avoid feeling deprived of the sight of the analyst. They may prefer visual connection to the analyst via a web camera at the beginning and end of each session. Some choose VOIP with web camera because they want to imagine the analyst looking at them. Some refuse because they do not want to be looked at when they cannot monitor the looking and the analyst's reactions, the same resistance as they would feel in person on the couch with the analyst out of view. Some do not want to be looked at because they want to hide their struggle, which is evident on the face, as if the face were the only sign of their distress.

On the telephone or on the Internet, the analyst deals with resistance expressed in forgetting to call, speaking softly, not using a headset, moving away from the microphone, accepting other calls, and chatting as if on a social call, in addition to silence, hesitation, coughing, lateness, non-payment, displacement and so on, often seen in in-person analysis when anxieties block the flow of associations. Analysts via telephone or via Internet observe the usual technique of maintaining a neutral position conceptualized according to their respective traditions as being equidistant between the generations: among ego, id, and superego; or among ideal object, rejecting object, exciting object, central ego, antilibidinal ego, and libidinal ego. They work with dreams and free association, sometimes more easily on the phone for those analysands who are inhibited by the bodily presence of the analyst. So although one area of exploration is hidden, another comes to the fore. As the sessions continue over time, the issues are revisited and worked through. Transference flourishes on the telephone as in real life, evokes a countertransference response from the analyst, and the transference-countertransference dialectic is analyzed as it would be in in-person sessions.

Reflections on telephone and in-person sessions: clinical example continued

After telephone analysis had been established for some months, the analyst learned that when Mr. M, the analysand I described earlier, was nine years old, his mother sent him for a couple of weeks to his aunt's house across the border in Canada. Mr. M perceived this as a punishment for his having witnessed and spoken about his mother's seduction by a powerful person at their synagogue, which resulted in a huge upheaval at home and the departure of her lover. Repeatedly at his aunt's, he was left with a male babysitter who, apparently unknown to the aunt, was sexually abusive. When the boy asked to call his mother to take him home, his aunt would not allow it until he cried and cried. Then it took many tearful calls before his mother accepted him home. He was vulnerable to sexual abuse because of the overstimulation and guilt around his mother's affair, and unable to speak about it because of the fear of causing more trouble. So neither aunt nor mother was told of the reason for his need to leave for home.

Mr. M's worry about calling in terror of the next abuse was recreated in difficulty calling his analyst, which he described as follows: "Perhaps I think my call to you for help will not be met or will be dismissed, or you will not understand that things are as bad as they are, when I actually think you get it. So, the telephone is my way out of my internal trauma, as it was with Arthur [the babysitter] – at least, that is the hope, but it seems to take many, many calls for this to happen. Just like it seemed I was with Arthur forever, it seems like it's taking a very long time to get through all this. I often wonder if you're there at the other end."

Falling silent on the phone reminded Mr. M of being unable to call his mother the time he was left in hospital for pneumonia. As he put it, "I couldn't talk much anyway, because my voice was weak. I feel this same feeling on the phone at times in my silence. Words are in my head, but I can't seem to get them out. While in the hospital, it felt like there was no way to reach my mother, partly because even when she was present, she seemed so absent."

Mr. M said that losing in-person sessions because of his move reminded him of the time he was sent away. "My mother may have had good intentions for my health in sending me to her sister, but I experienced it as being sent away because I wasn't the right child. My mother had a baby on the way by then, a girl, the right child. I felt like I was too much for her, which was part of the reason for being sent away. I was too sick, too quiet, too needy. I feel I am not a good patient – too sick – and not a good phone patient – too quiet, just like I felt with my mom. And I am afraid of being too much for you."

Mr. M was, if anything, even more anxious in person when he came to my office for a week of analysis approximately three times a year. He attributed that to having spent so much time in a doctor's office, and raising the fear that I, like that doctor, would send him to the hospital, a fear that became intense when I did refer him to a colleague in a large medical building for a medication consultation. "The travel required to your office may recreate those moments of travel to the doctor's office, which I simply dreaded, yet needed to stay alive. I also feel concern about you keeping the door locked. I fear being trapped on the outside (can't get in, like I couldn't with my mother's heart) and trapped on the inside so that I can't escape from harm. Being shut in your office with the double door is like being trapped with Arthur, especially when I feel tormented in your presence. At least on the phone, I feel a bit safer."

Mr. M noted that the analyst seemed more distant to him in person, and was puzzled as to why that was the case. He tried to explain: "It may be my experience of my mother as absent when present. It may be that the phone provides a kind of intimacy, a whispering in my ear, like a mother might do with a child. You just seem closer on the phone." In my office, he found my physical presence a mixture of reassuring and threatening, especially when talking about traumatic sexual material, which nauseated him. He said, "In your office, I find it embarrassing when I feel like I am going to throw up on your rug and we work on the feeling together, but over the phone there have been a couple of times when I actually did have to throw up, and hung up a few minutes early." At moments like these, the frame offered by analysis on the telephone could not fully contain the anxiety felt in the body. On the other hand, the use of the telephone allowed the analysand to reveal more vivid detail about sexual abuse than was possible in person and gave the body freedom to give full expression of fear and disgust. Hanging up the phone a few minutes early gave expression to the wish to remove himself from the analyst as a torturing figure.

Mr. M's childhood was punctuated by trips to the doctor and the hospital. Similarly, the in-person analysis was interrupted by telephone sessions, and the telephone analysis was interrupted by in-person sessions. For Mr. M, telephoning the analyst had multiple meanings: it was both reminiscent of being in the hospital and at the aunt's far from his mother whom he could not call, and also reminded him of finally reaching his mother and being listened to. The telephone was both the block to, and the means for recovery, but telephone analysis goes slowly as did the time the analysand spent as a child feeling frightened in the hospital and at his aunt's. Being in the office was reminiscent of being trapped in a hospital room, especially of the time he was in the oxygen tent, being shut in behind locked doors with a frightening babysitter, and also of being with a mother whose good attention is longed for.

Verbal and non-verbal communication in traditional and teleanalysis

Remote analysis by telephone is different from traditional or shuttle analysis in that the two bodies, analysand and analyst, are not together in the office, and the contact is primarily auditory. However, in both traditional analysis and teleanalysis, the analyst privileges conversation over bodily interaction: The body of the analysand is lying down in a state of reduced mobility so that action is not available as a discharge route, but in traditional analysis the body's non-verbal clues can be seen. The use of the telephone relies upon speech and analytic listening as the primary mode of exchange in psychoanalysis. Continuing in telephone analysis with a woman patient who had to move after a period of in-person analysis, Hanly (2007) learned that erotic elements of her transference were evoked because she could imagine him as a younger man without visual contradiction, and a dependent maternal transference (previously covered by a paternal transference in in-person sessions) was revealed due to hypercathexis of his calming voice. Indeed, without the libidinal presence of the body, the telephone privileges semiology of voice (Aryan et al. 2009).

Focusing on only the medium of speech, the analyst becomes more intent on listening. Working with a woman patient, Zalusky (2000) found herself "more present to hear the nuances of her associations" (p. 24). Finding that he listened more intently, Leffert (2003) said that "the treatment becomes an analysis of words and voice: the verbal comes to carry all the contact and interaction, replacing appearance and visual contact" (p. 117): It is a "hyperanalytic process" putting "everything into verbal utterances ... a central goal of any analysis" (p. 124). From clinical experience, we know that the unique form of a person's verbal expression signifies a great deal about that person's history, culture, and personality, and specific internal object relationships. From research we have learned that the adult attachment interview uses speech patterns to predict attachment style accurately (Main 1995). This sensitivity to the voice increases when the visual channel is blocked. The voice provides a substitute channel for understanding, through which the symptom comes alive to be worked with directly. As Freud put it, "while we are working at one of these symptoms we come across the interesting and not undesired phenomenon of 'joining in the conversation'" (Freud 1893, p. 296 fn, p. 37 fn).

Even though we cannot see the analysand in teleanalysis, and we must relate through the voice, the body joins in the conversation. This is illustrated in the analysis of Mr M, to which we now return.

In the mid-phase of treatment when Mr. M finally found the words to recount what actually happened when shut in the room where he was being terrorized by the male babysitter, he began to cough uncomfortably, and so did the analyst. The analyst thought at first that she was coughing in resonance with the boy's general anxiety about his safety, but then an image of gagging on a penis entered her mind and suggested a more specific source of her anxiety, possibly conveyed to her by projective identification. She felt embarrassed by being unable to speak for the benefit of Mr. M, because of trying to suppress the cough, the terror, and the specific image. Mr. M continued coughing almost to the point of vomiting, and in response to the analyst's telling him that she had the impression that he was trying to evacuate a traumatic image, he eventually found his words and told of the trauma of being forced to perform fellatio and then being too afraid to tell a parent who would not believe him. Mr. M understood the vomiting impulse as a wish to get rid of the ejaculate. The analyst recovered, and work continued, analyst and analysand reviewing what had just happened.

Mr. M said, "I guess it was the only way to convey what happened, which I had blocked from my mind. It only came forward for me at the moment it did for you. When you were incapacitated like that, it reminded me of my illness being too much for my mom. I couldn't orient myself, and it felt as though you couldn't either. I am worried about hurting you, worried that my stuff will get into you (as it did). I felt an absolute sense of desperation in the moment, and I had to struggle to breathe. When Arthur was abusing me, that struggle to breathe took the focus much more than what was happening sexually. I was always worried about surviving with him, like I am psychically at times with you."

Reviewing this sequence together, Mr. M and his analyst joined in understanding the horror of the event, the shame at being taken over by it, the wish to evacuate the sadistic object, and the longing for an empathic response, empathy having been absent not only at the time of the abuse but also for a moment in the session when the analyst was incapacitated. Without visual clues and without words, the anxiety of the moment had been clearly transmitted in eidetic form as a projective identification, received, and put into words.

The interacting unconscious mind in teleanalysis

In in-person sessions, the unconscious minds of analyst and analysand are interacting in the context of bodily presence where desire and abstinence are evoked and, driving the recall of infantile sexuality and early experience, give access to implicit memory behaviors (Sachs 2003, p. 29). However, in telephone or VOIP sessions, the analyst's tone of voice alone produces a bodily response in the analysand and vice versa. True, the analyst cannot see this bodily response, but uses other observations, such as hesitations, tearfulness, catches in the breath, and changes in tone that reveal so much more than words alone.

Having moved from the in-person experience to the telephone session, the analyst starts listening with an image of the person, sitting in the waiting room, entering the door of the office, lying on the couch, and later, leaving the office. The analysand has a corresponding image of the analyst in the analytic chair. These images endure in telephone sessions in which there are no non-verbal cues. As the session proceeds, the sound of the voice delivered through headphones or from speakers in the room, evokes an image colored by the relevant affect. The voice of the unconscious conveyed in association, affective tone, hesitation, slip, and silence conjures a sensation that conveys the analysand's internal situation. This is no different from in-person analysis where although the analyst is looking at an analysand lying on a couch in the present, in the mind's eye, the analyst sees that person in many different situations past, present, and future, here in the office and in outside life, as associations flow. We may think we have a single view of ourselves and our patients in space but many different images and spaces are encoded in the brain (Ferrari 2010). The past that is forgotten is constructed in the here-and-now of the session to arrive at a more complete narrative of the person's history (Faimberg 2009).

When one route of communication is blocked by working on the telephone, other routes compensate because of cross-modal channels of communication (Anderson et al. 2009). Unconscious communication can occur on auditory, visual, and sensory routes. Language is embodied in the resonating sensorimotor system: words stir emotions. A purely auditory communication on the telephone provokes a visual image in the listener that is then put into words, as it would be in traditional analysis. Comparing process notes from a traditional and a teleanalysis session from the same analysand, Mirkin (2011) could not tell which was which, and neither could my colleagues in a teleanalysis working group (Scharff 2011).

Teleanalysis: contraindications and indications

Teleanalysis is not always indicated. Several analysand-specific factors need to be assessed, such as the capacity for maintaining the alliance and sharing responsibility for the management of the setting. The presence of borderline features with current suicidal/self-harming risk; the need for medication (unless a local psychiatrist is willing to take medical responsibility for assessing risk, prescribing, and monitoring side-effects); and the presence of substance abuse unless sobriety is maintained, all represent potential risk factors that need to be very carefully assessed as they would be for traditional analysis. Each case needs to be considered on its own merits, but the lack of in-person oversight may mean that these factors amount to an overwhelming contra-indication to teleanalysis.

Teleanalysis, however, is possible – and may be even easier – for those analysands with a history of trauma-related dissociation, where shame and embarrassment about traumatic early experiences could be easily provoked by being "seen" by the analyst. In the analysis of "severely traumatized people, the telephone may allow a necessary space in which they can begin to tackle the fears associated with intimacy" (Zalusky 2005, p.111).

Practical factors are also important, such as whether analyst or analysand have uncorrected deafness or when either of them speaks too softly or indistinctly, or is too silent to sustain the connection.

Analyst-specific factors are also a consideration: Teleanalysis is not a good idea if the analyst is made anxious by lack of in-person sessions, cannot rely on visualizing the physically-absent analysand, and feels disconnected. Teleanalysis is indicated when analyst and analysand are confronted with a circumstance that impedes the continuation of an ongoing analysis because of travel for work, relocation, illness including phobia, and commitments that interfere with the analysand's commuting to sessions during the analyst's available hours. Teleanalysis is indicated for those living in another country even if there is no already established analytic process, provided the analyst has met the analysand in person to make the assessment, has established the alliance in a preliminary sense, and has received agreement for in-person sessions at suitable intervals.

Although the prior establishment of analytic process in person is preferable, Gelman (2001) has reported that analysis has started before meeting the patient who lives in a remote country, and Carlino (2011) has written that he foresees a day when teleanalysis might be preferred by digitally connected young people even though they live near an analytic center. Analysts in cities such as New York and Los Angeles with long, traffic-bound commutes are reporting that some patients are requesting telephone sessions. In any case, the practice of teleanalysis is still experimental, and so the analysand should be told this before consenting to teleanalysis, and the analyst is advised to consult with a group of colleagues who are gathering experience in this area for further study.

Experience with the clinical effectiveness of psychoanalysis using telephone or Internet has implications for expanding training opportunities for candidates in remote locations and for the spread of psychoanalysis. The question that teleanalysis then faces is whether it is functionally equivalent to an in-person analysis in terms of fostering dreaming, free association, resistance, and transference–countertransference experience of sufficient intensity to evoke in candidates having teleanalysis a conviction about the working of the unconscious, the formation of character defenses, and the interpretive skill to achieve therapeutic action, such that these candidates become effective analysts with their own analysands (Sachs 2009).

Training analysis by telephone or Internet may be authorized for candidates in exceptional circumstances. When training analysts across regions have accumulated experience in analysis by telephone or Internet, and research analysts have published their results on its clinical effectiveness, teleanalysis may some day be offered with confidence as an alternative or a supplement to condensed analysis for disadvantaged candidates, and so bring psychoanalytic training to remote locations. "We must change our way of looking at the use of the telephone if we are to provide truly patient-friendly analytic treatment and trainee-friendly analytic training" (Richards 2003, p. 32).

Conclusion

Of necessity, psychoanalysis is making increasing use of the telephone, videoconference, and VOIP in clinical practice and in teaching. Out of that necessity, teleanalysis finds an opportunity for opening up new pathways of understanding and extending the reach of psychoanalysis to new frontiers.

Some analysts believe that psychoanalysis, a professional art based on the harmonics of unconscious communication, augmented by technology cannot possibly transcend the limits of distance. Others note that unconscious communication and analytic process occur in telephone and VOIP analysis as they do in traditional in-person analysis. The deficit of losing the actual communication of physical presence has to be admitted, and the loss acknowledged. "By being sensitive to what we are losing, we help our patients be more open about their own feelings of loss" (Zalusky 2005, p.108). Then we are free to develop a heightened appreciation for unconscious communication via the transmission of sound. The objection that innovative telephone analysis is a seductive, fashionable, elastic practice that fails to interpret transference (Argentieri & Mehler 2003) may reflect the debate about various philosophies of psychoanalysis more than about telephone analysis itself (Zalusky 2003a).

Notes

1 Often referred to as Skype, the trade name of the major carrier, but here the generic term VOIP is preferred.

References

Anderson, G., Scharff, D., Scharff, J., and Symington, N. (2009). Telephone analysis. Panel on Telephone Analysis, International Psychoanalytic Congress, Chicago, August 2009.

Argentieri, S. and Mehler, J. A. (2003). Telephone 'analysis': 'Hello, who's speaking?' *Insight, 12*:17–19.

Aronson, J. K. (Ed.) (2000a). *The use of the telephone in psychotherapy*. Northvale, NJ: Jason Aronson.

Aronson, J. K. (2000b). Use of the telephone as a transitional space. In: J. Aronson (Ed.) *The use of the telephone in psychotherapy* (p.129–149). Northvale, NJ: Jason Aronson.

Aryan, A., and Carlino, R. (2010). Desafíos del y al psicoanálisis contemporáneo. Vicisitudes de lo establecido frente a lo nuevo que va surgiendo. El psicoanálisis telefónico. Unpublished paper VI APU. International Multidisciplinary Congress, Montevideo, Uruguay, August, 2010.

Aryan, A., Berenstain S., Carlino R., Grinfeld P., and Lutenberg, J. (2009). Psicoanálisis por teléfono. Panel on Telephone Analysis. International Psychoanalytic Congress, Chicago, August 2009.

Benaim, B. (2009). Personal communication.

Benson, R. M., Rowntree, E. B., and Singer, M. H. (2001). Final report of ad hoc committee on training analysis via telephone. Unpublished report to the Board on Professional Standards of the American Psychoanalytic Association.

Bollas, C. (2009). Personal communication.

Brainsky, S. (2003). Adapting to, or idealizing, technology? *Insight, 12*(1): 22–24.

Carlino, R. (2011). *Distance psychoanalysis*. London: Karnac.

Chodorow, N. (2004). Creating a physical surround in the absence of physical presence: Clinical observations on phone treatment. Unpublished paper. Vermont Association for Psychoanalytic Psychology, November 2004.

Faimberg, H. (2009). The past as resistance, the past as constructed. Unpublished paper. IPA Congress, Chicago, July 2009.

Ferrari, P. (2010). Understanding others through shared representations: The neural underpinnings of intersubjectivity. Keynote address at conference of the International Psychotherapy Institute, Salt Lake City, March 2010.

Freud, S. (1893). The psychotherapy of hysteria. *Standard Edition, 2*: 253–305.

Freud, S. (1912). Recommendations to physicians practicing psychoanalysis. *Standard Edition, 12*: 109–120.

Gelman, M. H. (2001). The use of the telephone in analysis: Therapeutic compromise or primary modality of treatment. Unpublished paper at the Sandor Ferenczi Conference in Budapest, Hungary, February 23, 2001.

Hanly, C. (2007). Case material from a telephone analysis. Unpublished panel presentation. Spring Meeting, American Psychoanalytic Association, Seattle, June 2007.
Leffert, M. (2003). Analysis and psychotherapy by telephone. *Journal of the American Psychoanalytic Association, 51*: 101–130.
Lindon, J. (2000). Psychoanalysis by telephone. In: J. Aronson (Ed.) *The use of the telephone in psychotherapy* (p. 3–13). Northvale NJ: Jason Aronson.
Lutenberg, J. (2011a). Presentación de material clínico del análisis telefónico. *Tratamiento psicoanalítico telefónico* (pp. 113–142). Lima, Peru: Siklos SRL.
Lutenberg, J. (2011b). Reflexiones técnicas a partir de las sesiones con Irene. *Tratamiento psicoanalítico telefónico* (pp. 143–186). Lima, Peru: Siklos SRL.
Main, M. (1995). Attachment: Overview, with implications for clinical work. In: S. Goldberg, R. Muir, and J. Kerr (Eds.) *Attachment theory, social developmental and clinical perspectives* (pp. 407–475). Hillsdale, NJ: Analytic Press.
Mirkin, M. (2011). Telephone analysis: Compromised treatment or an interesting opportunity? *Psychoanalytic Quarterly, LXXX*(3): 643–670.
Richards, A. K. (2003). Fruitful uses of telephone analysis. *Insight, 12*(1): 30–32.
Robertiello, R. C. (1972–73). Telephone sessions. *Psychoanalytic Review, 59*: 633–634.
Rodriguez de la Sierra, L. (2003). 'If it helps, why not?' *Insight, 12*: 20–21.
Sachs, D. (2003). Telephone analysis – sometimes the best choice? *Insight, 12*: 28–29.
Sachs, D. (2009). Far away, so close. Unpublished paper. Panel, International Psychoanalytic Congress, Chicago, July 2009.
Saul, L. J. (1951). A note on the telephone as a technical aid. *Psychoanalytic Quarterly, 20*: 287–290.
Scharff, J. S. (2010). Report of panel on telephone analysis. International Psychoanalytic Association Congress, Chicago, August 2009. *International Journal of Psycho-Analysis, 91*: 989–992.
Scharff, J. S. (2011). Findings of the International Working Group on teleanalysis. Precongress, International Psychoanalytic Association meeting, Mexico, August 2011. *Bulletin of the International Psychotherapy Institute, 15*(2): 2.
Snyder, E. (2011). The use of Skype in supervision. Panel, Winter Meeting, American Psychoanalytic Association, January 2011.
Varela, Y. (2007). Transference as a playground: Two analytic settings. Unpublished paper.
Yamin Habib, L. E. (2003). Physical presence – a sine qua non of analysis? *Insight, 12*: 25–27.
Zalusky, S. (1998). Telephone analysis: Out of sight but not out of mind. *Journal of the American Psychoanalytic Association, 46*: 1221–1242.
Zalusky, S. (2000). Telephone analysis. In: J. Aronson (Ed.) *The use of the telephone in psychotherapy* (pp. 15–43). Northvale, NJ: Jason Aronson.
Zalusky, S. (2003a). Adaptation or idealization of theory? *Insight, 12*(2): 34.
Zalusky, S. (2003b). Dialogue: Telephone analysis. *Insight, 12*: 13–16.
Zalusky, S. (2005). Telephone, psychotherapy and the 21st Century. In: M. Stadter M. and D. Scharff (Eds.) *Dimensions of psychotherapy: Dimensions of experience: Time, space, number, and state of mind* (pp. 107–114). London: Routledge.

Chapter 4

Psychic development in a virtual world

Florence Guignard

The globalization of virtual communication

Communication and social boundaries within Western society are changing at an ever-increasing rate. The extraordinarily rapid development of technology and its applications are partly responsible for this. Together with the more varied permutations in contemporary family units (e.g. single parent families) in which children are being brought up nowadays, the digital revolution has had a great impact on the development of mental functioning. This seems to be particularly relevant to children and young adults and can be observed in their social adaptation patterns. The virtual world inhabited by young people today is a second-generation phenomenon that is beginning to have a lasting effect. Every psychoanalyst has to take these issues into account.

The relationship between the individual and society is always changing. Contemporary Western society bears very little resemblance to the nineteenth-century Austrian society in which Freud grew up. Nowadays the development of the individual's mental life – the domain of psychoanalysis – has been pushed into the background by such considerations as efficiency and adaptability to the environment, which, in itself, has changed very rapidly over the past few decades.

The instantaneous transmission of information – and misinformation – anywhere in the world means that people have to deal with new kinds of demands on the economic aspect of their instinctual drives and, consequently, with new kinds of anxiety.

The globalization of virtual communication necessarily brings in its wake two main consequences: 1) an expectation for instantaneous fulfilment of wishes and desires, modelled on what happens in a virtual world, and 2) an increased risk that the three aspects of the basic assumption group mentality (Bion 1961) – fight/flight, pairing and dependence – will take over from thinking for oneself.

In my view, several more generations will pass before digital functioning becomes properly integrated in society. Meanwhile society will be influenced by it to a degree and in a direction that, in the short term, is impossible to estimate. What are we, as psychoanalysts, to think about such a situation?

Expanding psychoanalytic knowledge

As I shall develop below, the family-based society of the past centuries is now changing at a high speed. If we bring such a consideration together with that of the fast development of digital functioning, we must give some thought to the following question: Will the basic parameters of psychoanalysis adapt to this rapid evolution of society? Over the past 20 years there has been a significant change in the kinds of patients who contact a psychoanalyst in the hope of relieving their mental distress. No doubt the classical model of the neuroses, as described by Freud, applies to fewer and fewer patients; this would seem particularly to be the case in the younger and perhaps more complicated generations.

As the years go by we have come to realize that we are dealing more and more with 'borderline states'. Fragile and poorly structured, the frontiers between self and other, between thought and action, between internal and external reality and – more recently – between the real and the digital world, fragment more easily when the boundaries or limits set up by society have become more flexible, weak and confused.

These types of 'borderline' patients require us to reconsider more carefully the very *models* we have been referring to. It is quite legitimate to ask whether the aims of contemporary psychoanalysis are to deal with psychic structures, both individual and social, which are sufficiently similar to those Freud was analysing 100 years ago. Would the psychoanalytic *corpus* still be of any use – even after the relevant modifications – in our present-day explorations of the human mind? Such a problem involves a whole series of questions concerning the outcome of wishes, guilt, repression and identification. It also raises two further questions: 1) are *infantile neurosis* and *transference neurosis* fundamental, as they have been since 1905 when Freud published his seminal work in which he described his discovery of *infantile sexuality* and the part it plays in mental functioning, and 2) if they are not, what *elements* of these two concepts could contemporary psychoanalysts still regard as fundamental?

Freud's (1905) *Three Essays* is an essential point of reference because, if we do away with infantile sexuality, the very idea of psychoanalysis and the concept of neurosis become meaningless. This leads to another question: are the *status* and *modalities* of infantile sexuality as they operate on the development of mental life and psychopathology exactly the same today as they were in 1905?

If we do not want to be overwhelmed by those psychotherapists who pin all their hopes on behaviour modification techniques and on how to change conscious thinking processes, we psychoanalysts have to stop considering psychoanalytic theory as a kind of bedrock, but rather see it as a set of models, constantly called into question and re-formulated in order to take into account not only progress in method and modifications in technique but also the sociological changes that have occurred since psychoanalysis first emerged as a science. We should remember that Freud recommended to Ferenczi that theories should not be fabricated but that they should just 'fall into one's house as uninvited guests'.[1]

His Majesty the baby: a narcissistic object?

Children will feel the impact of 'virtual reality' most keenly. Given their emotional and intellectual immaturity, it is already difficult enough for children to establish a capacity for symbolization as a tripartite relationship: the ego, the symbol and the object symbolized. Children inevitably carry with them the hallmark of previous generations and their parents. In my opinion, however, there is a significant drift towards the Infantile in adults (Guignard 1995; 1996). As a strange historical/a-historical conglomerate, the crucible of primal fantasies and sensory motor experiences that can be stored as memory traces, the Infantile may be regarded as the psychic locus of the first, unrepresentable emergence of the drives. All that we can ever know of this 'advanced action' is its representable derivatives, in the form of infantile sexual theories on the one hand and memory traces on the other.

The Infantile is a basic structure on the fringes of our animal nature, the depository and container of our drives, be they libidinal or hateful on the one hand or epistemophilic on the other; it is that combination of drive related and 'flexible' structural elements that renders a person unique.

The notion of the Infantile is relevant to this particular discussion because even though, in theory, adults have the task of bringing up the younger generations, in practice they project more than ever into children their own infantile hedonism and, in so doing, satisfy it. What is missing here is an essential dimension of every civilization: a *latency period in space and time* between the formulation of a wish and its satisfaction.

These changes are brought about by various factors. Nowadays in the Western world children begin life in society at an early age: day nursery at three months, nursery school at three or even two years of age. Family life is reduced to a minimum for two main reasons: first, children spend little time at home and, second, the structure of families is being transformed. The extended family has been eroded in the child's actual neighbourhood, and grandparents nowadays are often still professionally active. In addition, given the way in which family life has evolved, children have to split their parental cathexes at an early age. Today the child's biological parents tend to live together for only a short period, if at all: they may eventually separate, with each of them restructuring his or her love life in 'reconstituted' families, either homo- or heterosexual – or, indeed, the mother may end up raising the child on her own. The paternal third-party role, which is essential if the infant is to break free from symbiosis (Bleger 1967) and set up a proper Oedipal configuration, is at risk of being sidelined or undermined in various ways, though this will depend on the mother's ability to keep the third in mind. In its place the social group, along with its basic assumption mentality, may then replace the contribution of the original parental couple.

When parents impose on their children such drastic – and often repeated – changes in life, they cannot avoid experiencing powerful guilt feelings, of which they may be more or less conscious. Some try to offset these feelings by giving their children a great deal in the way of material goods in the hope of easing the emotional deprivation that they are inflicting on them. In turn, the children soon learn to take advantage of the splitting that has been forced upon them, and play one side of their divided biological family against the other.

The erosion of latency, repression, and Nachträglichkeit

Freud's models of infantile and transference neurosis were originally based on his discovery that infantile sexuality developed in two phases, separated by what he called the latency period. The latter is devoted to the development of epistemic instincts and the construction of an ideal superego via acknowledging the difference between the sexes and generations. The acknowledgement of these differences also implies that the identification with the parents ensures the future supremacy of the reality principle over the pleasure/unpleasure principle.

However, I am suggesting that this description is now becoming obsolete in our society. From my day-to-day clinical work, and from my questioning of many practitioners of child and adolescent psychoanalysis over the past ten years in several European countries, I have come to think that the psychological development of children in our society has changed more in the past 15 years than it has at any time during the second half of the twentieth century. Effectively we are witnessing the disappearance of the latency period as defined by Freud in 1905.

The erosion of a latency phase has important implications. As mentioned before, this is a two-generations process that began around the 1970s, when psychoanalysts acknowledged that the difference between the sexes and between generations has been steadily blurred both in family relationships and in social ties. Once rid of the restricting-but-containing function of educational demands, the children of the *next* generation – that is the children of the 1970s generation – have had to find other defensive barriers against the growing power of the instinctual drives. Nowadays, these barriers are essentially group-based rather than family-oriented. In turn this gives rise to a new set of issues for society in general and for communication between individuals in particular. There is no longer any 'cooling down' of drive-related manifestations in children between six and 12 years of age; instead of deflecting their sexual drives towards sublimated activities, these 'latency' children are just as excitable as three- to five-year-olds in their 'Oedipal' phase. Hyperactivity as a syndrome is on the increase and brings in its wake new troubles of symbolisation (Salomonsson 2006). One important implication of these changes is that the concept of neurosis is no longer lying at the heart of the economic model of mental development.

Virtual reality and the principles of mental functioning

The speed of technological advance and means of communication modifies in a very profound and hitherto-unknown manner the feeling of solitude that human beings used to experience.

Virtual reality facilitates direct communication between any one individual and other people, who previously, for both geographical and sociological reasons, would have otherwise remained out of reach. In these virtual encounters the difference between the sexes and between generations no longer plays its traditional role. Anyone writing on the web can cheat and pretend to be what he/she is not. We know of many cases of abuse where children or adolescents – as well as adults – believe they are talking to a potential boyfriend or girlfriend when in fact his/her digital counterpart is totally inadequate, if not overtly perverse. The excitement linked to the speed of these exchanges tends to blur the ability to reflect on such a situation.

We know now that this vast domain of relationships has an impact on the network of closer ties represented by the child's family and social and school environment. The secret scent of virtual communication is all the more exciting for the child and/or the adolescent, as he/she becomes part of a team of innumerable 'friends'. Social networking sites disqualify the meaning of words such as 'friendship' and 'love'. Meanwhile, the child's *real* relationship with his/her *real* environment is left aside. We all know that any intimate relationship has to be 'nourished' by both partners. However, where parents are too busy and the children are too involved in their virtual relationships, there will be no psychic food for the development of the child's emotional life.

Clinical example: His educated and psychoanalytically-oriented mother brings Tim, a nine year old, to me, because of his depressive mood. During my first interview with him alone, Tim is kind and polite, but he doesn't speak much. He looks somewhat sad and dreamy.

I ask him: 'What are you thinking of?'

He hesitates, and then says: 'I am thinking of a game I have on my Playstation.'

I ask: 'What is this game about?'

He looks at me, very astonished, and starts explaining the game to me: you have to gather as many goods as possible and then you can exchange them with your 'partners'.

Tim accepted then to come and have regular psychotherapy sessions, because, as he said: 'I'd never imagined that you'd be interested in my games.'

Only after several months of psychotherapy did I suggest to Tim it might be possible to find partners in the close environment with whom he could exchange emotional food and goods.

This brief example illustrates how children take for granted their parents' disinterest in their virtual world. It is through being interested in what the virtual world offers to them – what it represents in their subjective experience – that it may then be possible to help children to consolidate actual embodied relationships without retreating defensively into a virtual world.

Another problem lies in the fact that virtual reality is predicated on a completely different relationship to the pleasure/unpleasure principle and to the reality principle than fantasy. Virtual reality offers an illusion of what is real, thus circumventing the need for mentally processing the links and transformations on which a healthy relationship between the inner mental world and external reality is based.

On the axis perception ↔ representation, virtual reality locates the cursor much closer to perception than to representation: it forces on the spectator a great amount of pre-digested perceptions, whose relationships to the real world are more or less out of kilter. Thus, the escape route it offers, when perceived reality is too painful, becomes all the more attractive. This situation appeals therefore to the child's passivity. We could think of it in terms of a 'narcissistic splitting of the self' (Ferenczi 1932) or a 'passive splitting' (Meltzer 1986) and we know that when passive splitting dominates secondary defence mechanisms such as repression, this plays a significant role in the breakdown of mental functioning – to such an extent that neurotic structures may disappear altogether.

Virtual reality is a world of simulation that does *not* deal with *uncertainty* (Guignard 1990): all the *aficionados* of video games highlight qualities such as the control and narcissistic enhancement that they offer. The kind of communication offered by virtual reality implies a greater cathexis of know-how and performance rather than of emotions and the development of thinking that results from this. Of course, virtual communication on social networking sites may also expose the individual to great uncertainty, for example, as to whether the other person will reply. On the whole, relationships are implicitly looked upon as a management issue, rather than as an aspect of one's personality development and of the quality of one's object relations. It is for these reasons that I am not persuaded that we can treat virtual space as if it were some kind of 'transitional space' – in fact I would like to go as far as to suggest that such an extension of the concept would not have been welcome by Winnicott.

Last, but not least, the development of an image-based universe that forces itself on visual perception completely changes the importance of, and the part played by, language in one's representation of the world. The world that is thereby offered to the conceptual apparatus is one of pre-digested visual perceptions, whose relationship to the individual's own internal objects are unknown and unimportant. As a result, it is very tempting for the individual to replace the internal mental world of representations linked emotionally to his or her internal objects with a universe of images that are forced upon visual perception. It follows that there is no need to develop any internal communication, since the part inner discourse plays in exploring the relationship with one's internal objects is similarly diminished.

The consequences for psychoanalytic treatment

I shall try to examine briefly, from three main perspectives, the consequences of the position I have outlined with respect to the psychoanalytic approach to children.

1) The phenomenological angle

The epistemic drives are no longer structured around a primal scene fantasy and wish to understand the knowledge that – in fantasy or in reality – the parental couple is deemed to possess; and beyond them, the history of human thought. Diverted by the development of virtual reality, these drives are mainly oriented towards action, with its necessary recourse to a binary-logic system of symbolic equations – or, to use Peirce's terminology, of indices and icons – replacing tripartite symbol-formation (Segal 1957). Binary logic, however, leads directly to the enactment of whatever solution is adopted. The individual is thus pulled back towards the primary level of the pleasure/unpleasure principle as Freud described it (Freud 1925): '"I should like to eat this', or "I should like to spit it out".'

This action-based solution, which bypasses and evacuates for the time being all anxiety about what is unfamiliar and death, can have several consequences: a) de-cathecting the enigma of the Sphinx – that is, linear time and the finite nature of human life – and replacing it with a hyper-cathexis of immediate action experienced as timeless; b) increased denial of the reality principle and, above all, denial of the reality of one's own death and c) myths about transformation and rebirth tend to give more importance to the technological aspect of change to the detriment of developing mental capacities.

2) The dynamic and economic aspects

The de-cathexis of inner mental life goes hand-in-hand with a pathology of repression and, consequently, with the disorganization of the two-stage development described by Freud in his model of infantile neurosis. What he called *Nachträglichkeit* (Freud 1915) is not built up in the same way, because in this new context infantile modes of sexuality remain continuously manifest from the normal Oedipal age until puberty. There is an unrestrained arousing of infantile genitality, characterized by imitation of adult sexuality – this is a direct expression of the denial of the difference between generations. In a sense, I am suggesting that children no longer have any proper childhood. What appears as hyper-maturity seems most of the time to be nothing but pseudo-maturity. Depressive affects are evacuated by means of hyper-activity that tends towards a kind of burnout or suicidal breakdown.

3) The topographical and structural dimension

Oedipal elements are no longer structured in terms of an Oedipus complex, just as castration elements are not organized into a proper castration complex. As a result, in young adults, the truly genital capacity of intimate relationship is replaced by the continuation of phallic and group values – always in pursuit of some exploit or other, in a voyeuristic/exhibitionistic mind-set.

Consequences for the clinical practice of psychoanalysis

The considerable increase of so-called 'borderline' patients means that there is an increasing number of non-neurotic people who cannot use 'good enough' secondary defences such as secondary repression, negation, displacement, etc. (Freud 1936). These individuals have to rely upon primitive psychic defences: splitting, denial, idealization and pathological projective identification (Guignard 1996).

This new orchestration of the constituent elements of mental functioning, together with the endemic use of the primary level of the ego's defences by virtual reality – while secondary level defences gradually melt away – exposes psychoanalysts to countertransference challenges as well as technical difficulties. Our capacity to use our countertransference may be the most precious tool we have in the analytical field and assists us in identifying certain aspects of our 'Infantile' state (Guignard 1996) whenever it resonates with that of our analysand's, whatever their actual age.

Blind spots in the countertransference

We can overcome more or less easily the analyzed barrier of our own repression and maybe even of our own splitting. Nevertheless, our inner world operates mainly on a neurotic level, that of our countertransference neurosis. It is that model that manages to transform our infantile sexual theories into what emerges as our implicit analytical theory. That will give rise to inescapable – but absolutely necessary – 'blind spots' in our countertransference (Guignard 2001). These blind spots will lead us to think, and perhaps even to *enact verbally*, in projective identification with whichever of the patient's internal objects proves to be the most active on the analytical stage at that point in time.

One of the defensive operations that is most frequently used, especially when we are faced with primitive defence mechanisms rather than with secondary repression, is what I call 'plug-interpretations' (Guignard 1996). In setting these up we make particular use of the analysand's personal history and the somewhat random representations we have of the real people who are actually part of that narrative, as well as our knowledge of theory – and, therefore, our own implicit analytical theory.

In other words, emergence of the drives in the patient arouses in the analyst an attempt to deny anxiety about death, the *primum movens* of mental development.

Now, if the principal aim of any analysis is to encourage symbolization in the patient, it could well be the case that our ability to identify with children of forthcoming generations might be unable to cope with the remarkable changes in their world vision, as the capacity for symbol-formation might have a less important role to play for generations to come than in the past, given the importance that the virtual universe has for them. In other words, our aim as psychoanalysts – helping to set up and to organize an internal mental life – may not be quite as *interesting* for future generations, focused as they are on the globalization of virtual images already prearranged.

Technical challenges

The globalization of the binary-logic system that underpins virtual imaging invites psychoanalysts to take another look at earlier research into the world of autism (Tustin 1972; Meltzer 1975; Haag 1985). The time has come for psychoanalysis to examine autism and its *Weltanschauung* without, of course, relinquishing its psychoanalytic parameters and Bion's theory of thinking (Bion 1962).

Nowadays, it is no longer enough to speak of 'psychotic aspects' of the personality, or of 'autistic barriers' in children and adolescents whom we still look upon in terms of classical neurotic development. We have to try to understand in depth what it is that, in the binary-logic universe of virtual reality, becomes such a powerful attractor for our young patients that they no longer need to accomplish the mental work of symbol-formation linked to the internalisation of the object and, ultimately, to processing the loss of that object.

Clinical example: Mary is a bright young woman in her early thirties when she consults me on behalf of 'a friend' – whose name or existence she never mentioned anymore in four years of treatment. During the first interview, she is sitting down and looking at me with a kind of fake smile, unable to utter a single word. I feel an important anxiety floating in the air, although she is totally unable to be in contact with it. Her demeanour could give the illusion of a well-behaved young woman who is attending a social event with polite boredom.

During several months I shall have to do the main part of the talking, until she will be able to name some part of what she feels and thinks.

Mary lost her mother a few months ago and did not feel nor express any sorrow about that loss, although she says very willingly that she truly loved her mother. The only child of a family whose father died long ago, Mary occupies an important role in the management of an engineering firm. She is highly gifted and qualified to create new models of software. She also spends most of her free time surfing on the web. She is thus chatting with a lot of people whom she rarely meets and in whom she quickly loses any interest. She tells me that she never regrets any rupture, whether in reality or on the web. There is no difference to her between the persons she meets in reality – concretely or on the web – and the characters of the games she is playing on her very sophisticated Playstation.

After a few months of psychotherapy – face to face – she resents the fact that she is more often in contact with her anxiety. She explains: 'Before I came here, I was able to forget the mere fact that anxiety existed. I only had to open my computer and start playing on it or chatting with any unimportant person. Now, I happen to miss my mother and it is immediately unbearable. It's your fault, you convinced me that I had feelings, and I don't even know whether this is true!'

(A pause) 'No, I know it is true, I just don't want to face these emotions, it's so frightening! The virtual world is much easier to deal with; you simply dismiss "them" when you begin to feel you might be longing for "them".'

If we still believe in the power of the 'talking cure' to integrate the patient's instinctual drives, we must above all take a closer look at the pathology of *primary sadism*, the foremost expression of the fusion of the life and death drives (Klein 1927). As an offshoot of that early form of drive fusion, the structure of oral and anal sadism is *the* locus in the child's mental apparatus upon which drive organization of the adult world will exert its influence. That too is where the world of virtual reality may offer an omnipotent and Manichaean escape route to our young patients.

In addition, given the absence of any real latency period, child analysts must nowadays learn to grasp the micro-shifts of *Nachträglichkeit* as they take place within the psychoanalytic setting. In order to do so, the analyst may need to give special attention to 'the history of the treatment' in place of the 'history of the patient'. He/she should make use of the ground of their common memories whenever they give way to a second look upon the transference/countertransference relationship or any symptom that has previously been worked through by the analytical couple. He/she should not hesitate to take the first step and say, for instance: 'You remember the dream you told me about some time ago (or the play you had organized) where such and such happened? Well, couldn't we say that it resembles what you draw (or play) just now? As if you unwillingly repeated something that has to be understood. But I also see a difference (or several) between the two events (dreams, drawings, etc). Can you see it?' And so on.

Conclusion

The views I have outlined in this chapter are the outcome of my clinical observations and discussions with colleagues working primarily with children. I have suggested that the family-based society of our grand-grandparents is unlikely to reappear in a close future. Children's hyper/pseudo-maturity will probably go on developing more and more as years go by and parents may remain very 'infantile' in their attitude. Through their own parental identifications, the new generations are at risk of enhancing the priority given to hedonism and to the use of primary processes in the management of reality.

In vulnerable children digital reality could reinforce the idealization of action over reflection and of surface relationships that bypass the otherness of the other and preclude the development of enduring relationships.

Nowadays, sociologists make the distinction between the generations born from 1995 onwards and the previous ones: The younger ones are called: 'inborn digital users' and the older ones are defined as 'immigrant digital users'. No doubt nowadays children are the 'inborn' whereas most of us are the 'immigrant' users.

We have to do our best to adapt ourselves to this new country of human intelligence, but we also have to be careful not to lose our identity and our cultural patrimony. Metapsychology is part of that patrimony insofar as it is a description of how the human mind is managing its drives, emotions, relations and identity in certain conditions of culture and education. However, child analysts will be the first to discover the mental structures that today's children – tomorrow's adults – set up in lieu of the infantile neuroses with which they have been familiar. This is an opportunity that most certainly must not be missed. We shall have to refine our means of observation and in particular make full use of those elements of psychoanalysis developed by the successors of Freud's pioneering work. In my view, 'concepts of a third type' such as Klein's 'depressive position' and Bion's 'container/contained relationship' can still be useful landmarks for us in our everyday practice: the threat of a complete breakdown weighs more and more heavily on the individuals of the forthcoming generations, because contemporary society does not offer very much in the way of psychic containment. In turn, our present society might be at risk of breaking down, as the individuals that compose it do not take care of their common values anymore.

Nevertheless, if we are to maintain our thinking and understanding at their optimal level, we shall have to put on hold the neurotic model as a paradigm of normality, and resist the temptation to call a halt to our ongoing research by simply replacing it with another model that we know would diminish our anxiety.

We cannot change our way of doing things – we can never stop ourselves from cathecting the internal world of the mind that, for us, is the very material on which our work is based. To that end, we must show sufficient interest and flexibility in the virtual reality scenarios that our child patients put before us, so that the 'inanimate objects' of which they are composed may acquire 'a soul' (Lamartine 1826). That is the price to pay if these objects, no longer treated as prefabricated, are to be transformed into representations of the emotions rather than used as evacuative procedures.

Notes

1 Letter from Sigmund Freud to Sandor Ferenczi, 31 July 1915, three days after he had sent to Ferenczi the manuscript of 'An Overview of the Transference Neuroses' (Freud 1985a [1915]).

References

Bion, W. R. (1961). *Experiences in Groups and Other Papers*. London: Tavistock.

Bion, W. R. (1962). 'A Theory of Thinking'. *International Journal of Psycho-Analysis*, *43*: 306–310.

Bleger, J. (1967). *Symbiosis and Ambiguity: The Psychoanalysis of Very Early Experience*. London: Process Press.

Ferenczi, S. (1932). 'Confusion of Tongues Between the Adult and the Child', in: M. Balint (Ed.) *Final Contributions to the Problems and Methods of Psychoanalysis* (156–167). London: Karnac.

Freud, S. (1925). Negation. *Standard Edition*, *19*: 233–239.

Freud, A. (1936). The Ego and the Defence Mechanisms. *Writings*, *2*: 1–176.

Freud, S. (1985a [1915]). *A Phylogenetic Fantasy: An Overview of the Transference Neuroses*. Cambridge, MA: Harvard University Press.

Guignard, F. (1990). 'Devenir Adulte? Apprendre l'Incertitude', in: A-M. Alléon and S. Lebovici (Eds) *Devenir Adulte?* (pp. 123–141). Paris: PUF.

Guignard, F. (1995). 'The Infantile in the Analytical Relationship'. *The Institute of Psycho-Analysis, IJP*, 76(6): 1083–1092.

Guignard, F. (1996). 'Un Trouble de Pensée sur la Métapsychologie'. *Revue français Psychanalyse, 60*: 1551–1565.

Guignard, F. (1996). 'The Infantile in the Analytical Relationship.' *The Institute of Psycho-Analysis, IJP,* 76(6): 1083–1092.

Guignard, F. (2001). 'Le Couple Mentalisation – Démentalisation, un Concept Métapsychologique de Troisième Type'. *Revue français. Psychosomatique*, (20): 115–135.

Haag, G. (1985). 'Psychothérapie d'un Enfant Autiste' ['The Psychotherapy of an Autistic Child']. *Approche psychanalytique de l'autisme,* (3): 65–78.

Klein, M. (1927). 'Criminal Tendencies in Normal Children', *British Journal of Medical Psychology*, 7: 177–192. (Reprinted [1975] The Writings of Melanie Klein, Vol. I [pp. 170–186]. London: Hogarth Press.)

Lamartine, A. de (1826). *Milly ou la Terre Natale* [Milly, or the Land that Gave Me Birth]: 'Objets inanimés, avez-vous donc une âme Qui s'attache à notre âme et la

force d'aimer?' ['Inanimate objects, have you then a soul / That attaches itself to our own and forces it to love?']
Meltzer, D. (1986). *Studies in Extended Metapsychology*. Perthshire: Clunie Press.
Meltzer, D., Bremner, J., Hoxter, S., Weddell, D. and Wittenberg, I. (1975). *Explorations in Autism*. Perthshire: Clunie Press.
Salomonsson, B. (2006). 'The Impact of Words on Children with ADHD and DAMP'. *International Journal of Psycho-Analysis*, *87*(5): 1029–1047.
Segal, H. (1957). 'Notes on Symbol Formation'. *International Journal of Psycho-Analysis*, *38*: 391–397.
Tustin, F. (1972). *Autism and Childhood Psychosis*. London: Hogarth Press.
_______ (1981). *Autistic States in Children.* London: Routledge.
_______ (1986). *Autistic Barriers in Neurotic Patients*. London: Hogarth Press.

Chapter 5

An order of pure decision

Growing up in a virtual world and the adolescent's experience of the body

Alessandra Lemma

In our advanced technological culture the 'postmodern' body is sustained by fantasies of re-arranging, transforming and correcting, fuelling fantasies of limitless improvement and change. More specifically the body is there to be transcended rather than accepted as a cornerstone of reality. So-called 'progress' fuels the fantasy that we can exist, to borrow Ewald's (1993) telling phrase, in an "order of pure decision".

In this chapter I want to focus on one particular kind of technological development – the domain of cyberspace – and to consider the fate of the body in cyberspace. More specifically I will explore how cyberspace may be used by *some* young people as a way of bypassing the psychic implications of being-in-a-body and the related anxieties, which become prescient during the adolescent process. This focus may help us to understand some clinical presentations during adolescence where the young person is referred with so called 'addictions' to cyberspace and where anxieties rooted in the body – sometimes specifically focused on its appearance – may not be apparent at first assessment.

During adolescence, when the wish to transcend the body is often at its peak for some young people, the desire to be somewhere other than *in* a real body finds a receptive space in virtual worlds where the body is superfluous, and where mastery, control and the denial of otherness can be exploited. Immersion in cyberspace may then allow the young person to create "synthetic worlds" (Baudrillard, 1988) in which the body can be dispensed with, history is frozen and thinking is anaesthetised, affecting the capacity to manage conflict and pain in reality. This is not, *per se*, a new argument (see, for example, Wood, 2006; Curtis, 2007; Gibbs, 2007; Toronto, 2009).

In approaching this subject my aim is not to demonise the virtual domain. It is all too easy to come across as a Luddite if one invites a moment's reflection on the very real progress made possible by technological development (Robins & Webster, 1999). From a psychological point of view, it has been suggested that cyberspace may even be construed as a kind of transitional space that facilitates helpful experimentation with 'new' identities (Turkle, 1995, 2005; Allison et al., 2006; Dini, 2009), and that the imaginary possibilities afforded by cyberspace can be used therapeutically (Suler, 2008). And yet, it is also the case that the techno environments of cyberspace are particularly receptive to the projection and acting out of unconscious phantasy, and like all 'good' things they may be put to less good use.

I will start by describing how virtual space can lend itself to being used as a psychotic enclave that can become especially compelling for vulnerable adolescents due to the demands made on the mind by the physical changes of puberty. Through detailed clinical material of work with an adolescent girl and boy respectively, I will then illustrate how virtual spaces allow the individual to manage confusion and distress about the real body. Here, the self's integrity is sustained through pseudo-representations of the body that are defensively experienced in terms of 'play' rather than pathology, and that create obstacles to the invitation by the analyst to reflect on the function of cyberspace in the individual's experience, especially of being-in-a-body.

The seductions and perils of technological embodiment

Cyberspace[1] refers to a computer-generated space that is viewed by the participant and responds to the stimuli from the participant. Virtual reality is populated by a range of cybernetic automatons that provide the individual with a high degree of vividness and total sensory immersion in the artificial environment. Movements in virtual reality are the same as movements in physical reality: for example, one can fly or go through walls since the material constraints of the body do not apply. Importantly many of the games that can be played in virtual reality also make it possible to assume new identities and to create whole 'new' worlds. Massively Multiplayer Online Role-Playing Games (MMORPGs), for example, are highly dynamic and interactive to the extent that the player can feel as if living inside an alternative reality where it is possible to control how characters look, how they behave, what they do and what they say, all with a staggering degree of specificity.

Cyberspace is indeed imagined by its supporters as a zone of unlimited freedom with no restrictions. When the pursuit of such unlimited freedom becomes compelling and all consuming, this comes at a price because one important consequence of immersion in cyberspace is the corresponding shrinking of public space, and hence the loss of actual, physically mediated relationships that provide a kind of psychic anchor – an anchor that is particularly important during the tumult of adolescence. This is especially so for some vulnerable young people who may view withdrawal away from relationships mediated by physical presence as the only solution to their troubled internal and external relationships.

Because cyberspace forms part of the technologised landscape that is now a standard part of daily life across the world, this makes it easier, sometimes less conspicuous, for it to be deployed by some young people as a refuge away from the demands of the reality of embodiment and its particular meaning for them. Immersion in cyberspace can be used to bypass the arduous psychic task required to represent experience, giving way instead to simulation with the attendant risk that the 'fake' can replace the real and become more compelling.

Of course, there are many ways one can escape from the body, for example, through intellectual pursuits. The question of why some young people might become defensively 'bookish' while others turn to cyberspace is unlikely to yield any simple answers, but unlike immersion in intellectual work, immersion in cyberspace, because of its very particular qualities (see below) can accede more immediately to a state of disembodiment. This more immediate freedom from being-in-a-body and the omnipotence it promotes can be intoxicating for some. In this respect it is not dissimilar to taking drugs, with one important difference, however: computers are available everywhere nowadays and their use is socially sanctioned, whereas drug taking remains less accessible to many young people, is illegal and is not generally culturally sanctioned.

This begs the question of whether the widespread availability of the Internet gives form to new pathological manifestations, or whether it merely aids the enactment of particular self-object representations (see Dini, 2009). My own clinical experience makes me sceptical of the view that the Internet *per se* 'causes' psychological problems. Rather, I am suggesting, it provides a culturally reinforced and readily accessible vehicle for the enactment of conflicts related to our embodied nature that some adolescents are especially primed for given their developmental histories. This is consistent with evidence – sparse though it is – that those individuals who misuse the Internet, for example, have pre-existing problems (Morahan-Martin, 2008).

Research in this area, however, is plagued with conceptual and methodological difficulties, not least the absence of agreement over what constitutes 'Internet abuse' and if it should even be considered a disorder. What is clearer is that particular psychological factors are associated with excessive use of various kinds of virtual reality, such as loneliness (Whang et al., 2003), low self-esteem (Yang & Tung, 2007) and shyness and social anxiety (Pratarelli, 2005). There is also evidence to suggest that depressed young people are more likely to use the Internet more than a non-depressed group (Ybarra et al., 2005). Research also suggests that socially anxious and lonely individuals are more likely than others to develop a preference for online social interaction versus face-to-face (Ervin et al., 2004), which is an important predictor of Internet abuse (Morahan-Martin, 2008). The links with anxiety, shyness and depression are unsurprising given that avatars, for example, allow for the regulation of intimacy although, paradoxically, through creating the illusion of control over what the other sees and knows about the self, individuals often end up revealing more of themselves through this medium. This can sometimes have adverse consequences.

What this research also makes clear is that the young people who seek refuge in virtual worlds do not necessarily do so because they struggle with their bodies or have body image problems. The compulsive use of cyberspace is over-determined, and may be driven by different conflicts, but my focus in this chapter is restricted to understanding those clinical presentations where this misuse is in the service of managing a disturbing experience of 'otherness' that is felt to be concretely located in the body. Where this is the central unconscious preoccupation, I am suggesting that cyberspace is ideally suited to being defensively used to bypass the psychic implications of an embodied self. This may be understood as partly a function of some of cyberspace's specific features, as follows:

1. *It denies corporeality*: cyberspace defies the history, the transience and, indeed, the very physicality of the body. The exhilaration of virtual existence and experience comes from the sense of transcendence and liberation from the material and embodied world. The limitations and history of the physical body are thus suspended and may be disavowed. This presents the individual with the illusion of limitless possibilities – an 'order of pure decision'.
2. *It abolishes the reality of difference and separateness*: it achieves this in two ways:
    a. By promulgating the illusion of a disembodied self, the tyranny of the specular image need not apply in virtual space: we are all just bits and bytes. Virtual reality thus promotes the fantasy that despite differences, we are 'all the same really'. It is this promise of *sameness* that makes it so compelling for some young people because it bypasses any exposure to an experience of difference, and the sense of insufficiency we all have to find ways of managing in ourselves. In virtual reality, however, the promise of sameness with an ideal (as projected into an avatar, for example) is forever such that the painful awareness of the given body and of bodily separateness may be sidestepped.
    b. Through circumventing the reality of geographical boundaries, physical presence is no longer required to initiate or sustain a relationship as bodily presence is converted into pseudo-presence (Zizek, 2004). The reality, and I would argue the *necessity of distance*, and separation (Josipovici, 1986), are replaced by immediate communication bypassing the otherwise painful psychic work required to allow for the mourning of the absent or lost object. Instead, the thrill of speed substitutes for the reality of a real 'other' who cannot be ever fully controlled by the self.
3. *It suspends the history of the subject*: and hence the link to the anchor of the past is eroded, especially as it is recorded in the body. Multiple identities, like the Windows programme, can be opened and closed at will.

We have, effectively, the creation of what Raulet (1991) has referred to as "floating identities". This could conceivably have some constructive uses if a more positive experience of a 'new' self in cyberspace can be integrated with life 'offline' (Turkle, 1995; Allison et al., 2006). But where this kind of integration is not possible, the potential for pathological splitting is considerable.

4. *It promotes the illusion of interpersonal transparency*: we can enter a world where there are "no zones of disorder or darkness", as Foucault (1980) put it. The strangeness and opacity of the other is circumvented because the other is effectively the self's creation. Here the object – who is also disembodied – can be fully known and hence possessed (Arias et al., 1990; Gibbs, 2007).
5. *It encourages the use of mimetic defences and the development of imitative identifications*: which are primitive in nature and based on an appropriation of the other through imitation. As Gaddini (1969) has observed, imitation precedes identification. Such imitations are fantasies of being or becoming the object. The aim is *to become the ideal*, and not simply to strive to *be like it*, as we would expect if a more ordinary identificatory process were at work. This is especially apparent in those virtual games where people can look like and 'become' someone else according to their own specifications.
6. *It alters the relationship between internal and external reality*: because it offers an illusion of what is real, thus bypassing the need for the psychic work necessary for understanding that inner and outer reality are linked instead of being either equated or split off from each other. In the virtual world the psychic equivalence mode of reality (Fonagy & Target, 1996) dominates whereby the internal world that is projected into virtual space is seen to correspond to external reality. The technological environment of cyberspace thus confuses the boundaries between internal and external worlds, creating the illusion that internal and external reality are isomorphic. In these conditions of existence there are no limits to what can be imagined and acted out. As the self becomes intoxicated with omnipotence, it loses all contextual referents – of which the body is one – that would otherwise lend meaning to experience. Thinking is attacked: as fantasy and reality collapse into each other, there is no space from which to reflect. Virtual space may thus be seen as providing a psychic reserve within which all wishes are gratified as reality becomes an irrelevance (Wood, 2006). As Freud put it:

> The hermit turns his back on reality and will have no truck with it. But one can do more than this: once can try to recreate the world, to build up in its stead another world in which its most unbearable features are eliminated and replaced by others that are in conformity with one's own wishes.
>
> (1930:81)

The virtual world provides the kind of possibility Freud alludes to, allowing the individual to reclaim the infantile illusion of omnipotence.

The body in adolescence

The features of virtual space that I have outlined may become especially salient and compelling for those young people who struggle to adjust to the psychic demands imposed by the reality of the changing body that puberty forces upon them.

Anyone working with adolescents will recognise the importance of the body in mental life. Understanding the individual's experience of his *body-self* is indeed fundamental to understanding psychic structure across the lifespan (Rey, 1994). That the body is the starting point of mental functioning was core to Freud's (1923) own understanding of the development of the ego and he cemented the view, later developed by others, that the body-self is the container and foundation for the sense of self (Schilder, 1950; Winnicott, 1966, 1972; Mahler & Furer, 1968; Hägglund & Piha, 1980; Haag, 1985; Krueger, 1989; Sandler, 1994). One important implication of this is that the ego derives its functioning from body models (Lichtenberg, 1978), such that the earliest experiences of taking into the mouth (i.e. introjecting) and of spitting out (i.e. projecting) could be said to form the foundation of all experience (Abraham, 1924; Fenichel, 1945). Importantly, it is the foundation for a stable relationship to reality (Lichtenberg, 1978).

Freud thus understood that psychic development is rooted in the body, and consequently he emphasised the measure of the demand for work imposed on the psyche due to its link with the body. Given that the body is a basic fact of life that supports all other psychic functions, when it is denied functioning in all domains (emotional, cognitive and social) it can be severely impaired.

Throughout life the body is an arena of a potentially terrifying lack of control. The body is disturbing because it always bears the trace of the other. This fundamental psychic truth has to be somehow integrated into our image of ourselves (Lemma, 2010). Facing the reality of the body thus involves a paradox: it means simultaneously taking ownership of the body, its desires and limitations, *and* integrating the fact that the body is the site where we meet the other, where we negotiate the meaning of sameness and difference, of dependency and separation. The extent to which the body may then be felt to be a hospitable or inhospitable home for the self will reflect the quality of the earliest identifications.

At nodal developmental points, such as at puberty, we need to construe a new representation of the body to accommodate the changing body. Schilder (1950) stressed that the body image is structured by psychological, not anatomical requirements. Indeed, the psychic/libidinal map of the body is organised not just by the laws of biology, but also by the meanings and fantasies about the body. It is in fact more apt to say that we are dealing with an imaginary anatomy: out of the early experience of body states and physical exchanges with others we develop a representation of our body that is more or less enduring, and that contains both perceptual and evaluative components.

In order to underline what I consider to be the dynamically unconscious dimension of the representation we have of our bodies at any point in time, I prefer to use the term *body imagining(s)*[2] in the sense that the internal representation we have of our body is always of a fantasised body. This term thus more accurately denotes the potential fluidity in our body image, while also underscoring that the representation of the body in the mind is an unconscious psychic organisation powered by particular fantasies of the self-in-interaction-with-an-other. The body imagining – as I am defining it here – is therefore built on projective and introjective mechanisms. Importantly, this representation of the body is fundamentally a function of libidinal cathexes.

The period of adolescence has been described by several authors as involving an identity crisis (Blos, 1967; Erikson, 1968), but this requires some qualification: the psychic process of adolescence typically sets in motion an unsettling review of personal identity that is *rooted in the body*. Whereas at birth the mind may be said to develop from the body, in adolescence the body presents itself forcefully to the attention of the mind (Ferrari, 2004). Erections, masturbation and menstruation intrude into an oasis of relative calm in the physical domain characteristic of the pre-pubertal stage. For many young people the experience of an orgasm becomes a focal point around which a sense of reality of the genital can be further organised, accompanied by a sense of volitional control in the seeking of sexual satisfaction.

At the best of times, puberty initiates a complicated and unsettling internal process: the physical changes that trigger changes in the body image and hence in self-representation are also accompanied by changes in relationships with others – these changes are, in my view, inextricably linked and impact reciprocally on each other. The demands made by this inevitable developmental transition can simply be too much to bear for some young people (Laufer & Laufer, 1984; Bronstein, 2009; Flanders, 2009). For some development and change may be experienced as "catastrophic" (Bion, 1970). This is all the more so where the quality of the early relationships have contributed to a fragile, undercathected bodily self, or to entrenched splitting such that body parts may have become identified with bad, terrifying objects. In these cases an internal or external organ can be experienced as an alien object residing within the body rather than as an integrated part of the body-self. Body sensations may then need to be kept separate from the image of oneself as sexually mature.

Meltzer refers to the 'confusional anxiety' that he regards as typical for all adolescents:

> The confusion centres on their bodies and appears with the first pubic hair, the first breast growth, first ejaculation and so forth. Whose body is it? In other words, they cannot distinguish with certainty their

> adolescent state from infantile delusions-of-adulthood induced by masturbation with attendant projective identification into internal objects.
> (1967: 98)

Laufer (1968) echoes the question of ownership of the body that is latent in so many clinical presentations during adolescence: is it felt to belong to the young person or to the mother? In their detailed work on adolescence, Moses and Egle Laufer (1984) have highlighted the need to change the relationship to the body as the key task of adolescent development. Its outcome, they suggest, determines the final sexual identity on which the sense of self is based. As a result of the bodily changes due to puberty the young person must now integrate into his sense of who he is the reality of the mature sexual body. This is inextricably tied to the resurgence of primitive anxieties about dependency and separation from parental figures, and of Oedipal conflicts.

When there have been deficits in the baby's earliest relationship with the mother and her body, this will compromise his relationship to his body, and hence to reality. By the time of puberty, the adolescent's fantasies related to his new body can become profoundly disturbing. The young person may fear losing control over his body and mind. This may lead them to experience the body as the persecutor that has to be attacked. It is not just that the young person has to manage the reality of a body that can now actualise sexual and aggressive, conscious and unconscious fantasies; he is also confronted with the reality of separation from the mother's body.

Under the pressure of puberty, the young person who has not established a secure, positively cathected body imagining will struggle to manage the reality of his separate and differentiated body in relation to the Oedipal couple. Instead there may be a need to create an idealised body imagining, charged with omnipotent fantasies that sustain an experience of fusion or union with the idealised pre-sexual body of the mother. It is only when the young person can feel identified with the mother's body that he can reassure himself against the threat posed by separation. This can then result in a disavowal of the reality of the sexual changes and a marked splitting off of the body (Laufer & Laufer, 1984).

Clinical illustrations

The case examples that now follow are not intended to demonstrate that the availability of the Internet caused these young people's problems – I do not believe this to be the case, as I mentioned earlier; rather, I hope they illustrate how for them, immersion in cyberspace became their solution to an inner turmoil that was connected with their respective experiences of being-in-a-body. Both cases may be read as illustrations not just of how cyberspace can provide a means for escaping from the body, but also from thinking and feeling, which of course it does. This therefore requires clarification of the conceptual framework that guides my work and understanding of these clinical presentations, namely that a) body and mind are inseparable, b) that the body, developmentally speaking, is the first stimulus to thought, and that it continues to be so throughout life to varying degrees, and c) that the capacity for emotional intimacy and the capacity to establish and enjoy physical intimacy (not just in a sexual sense, but more broadly conceived as encompassing sensuality) are closely connected. Escaping the reality of the body thus invariably also entails an escape from a place in the mind where thinking and feeling are possible, and hence from where relating to the other as 'other' is also possible.

A virtual body floating in psychotic space

Sharon was 17 when I first met her in the context of a public health setting. She was referred because she hated her appearance and she was impaired in several aspects of her functioning. On presentation she fulfilled diagnostic criteria for Body Dysmorphic Disorder, and she was evidently severely depressed.

Sharon came from a relatively deprived socio-economic background. As far as she was concerned it was only the lack of finances that presented an obstacle to seeking cosmetic surgery: if she had the financial means she was clear that she would pursue it to obtain for herself what she fantasised to be a 'normal' and desirable body. Perhaps because she could not find a solution to her intolerable predicament through cosmetic surgery, Sharon turned to cyberspace instead. In cyberspace it was possible for her to sustain the fantasy of complete control over her self-presentation. As I will go on to illustrate, I understood this as her way of managing the profound paranoid anxieties she felt when in touch with the reality of her body and what it unconsciously represented.

Sharon was the eldest of two. Her parents lived together but their relationship was a violent one. Sharon said that she hated her father. She felt closer to her mother even though she experienced her as very inaccessible. The mother was often at home but she was severely depressed and found her own comfort through overeating. As a younger child Sharon had struggled to attend school and had spent long stretches of time at home with her mother. Throughout her life she had been anxious to maintain physical proximity to her mother and to be desired by her, but invariably she was left feeling that she could never enliven or impress her. Sharon believed that her mother was more invested in her younger brother.

Sharon described feeling ugly for as long as she could remember, but this feeling took hold in a particularly vicious manner around the age of 13. Menstruation had felt deeply unsettling and she had hated this moment in her life. Around this time she said that her face also erupted in acne. Since then she had been especially concerned about her skin and the shape of her face.

Her skin, she said, was now still blotchy and uneven. She could not say what was wrong with her face except that it was the "wrong shape", that somehow it was "too big". She was, in fact, an attractive girl with exceptionally smooth skin, as far as I could see. Yet she spent several hours every morning applying make-up and changing in and out of various outfits before she felt able to leave the house, which was not often. This led her to drop out of college and to disengage from her peer group.

She spent long periods of time at home, lying in bed, playing games on a small Nintendo, or she would sit at a computer and immerse herself in a range of virtual games where she acquired a new identity and new friends – a new life, in short. She created different characters and was especially concerned with their physical presentation. When she discussed this in therapy it was clear that she felt relieved and comforted by the transformations she underwent in her mind as she identified with her avatars, especially because she could imagine herself in a different and more desirable body.

Sharon spent numerous hours (often seven hours or more) every day mostly playing different games, but sometimes also visiting online chat rooms. She had one sexual relationship, aged 16, but this had left her feeling that sex was "overrated" and that she was not going to bother with it. Her account of a desultory sexual encounter was filled with shame and fear that she evidently needed to distance herself from.

It was hard to think with Sharon about her use of cyberspace. She dismissed what I said as irrelevant since the games were "just a bit of fun". The relationship Sharon developed with the computer itself was also important and similarly hard to think about. Interestingly, she was very possessive of the computer. Since she had to share it with the whole family, not least with her brother, access to it was often a source of heated rows. She described to me the way she enjoyed the feel of the mouse in her hand, and the pleasure she gained when she clicked and saw things happen on the screen, as if the responsiveness of the screen to her touch evoked a feeling of fusion with, and hence control over, the idealised maternal object that the computer, I thought, and the privileged space it gave her access to, had become identified with in her mind.

Her descriptions of online relationships were revealing: once she rather excitedly told me about a girl with whom she regularly 'chatted', but whom she had never met: "I know everything about her – I even know when she goes to the toilet!" This statement provided an important insight into one of the appeals of this kind of relationship: this disembodied other, about whom she paradoxically knew intimate physical details, was felt to be entirely transparent, knowable and accessible. For Sharon this encapsulated the enmeshed relationship she wanted to create with her mother. It expressed the fantasy of getting right inside her body (she would even know her bowel movements).

Sometimes Sharon missed sessions because she had been on the computer and 'forgot'. When we would explore this it became clear that she had been immersed in one of the games. When she was playing or online she entered a state of mind that was completely disconnected from reality: time ceased to matter and 'real' others ceased to exist. She felt very involved in her games and hated intrusions into this idealised space: she responded angrily if either of her parents interrupted her and asked her to do something. I knew, too, that she felt angry with me for intruding into this space through my invitations to think with her about how she used cyberspace. These incursions into her cocoon gave way to rages as she felt brutally pulled away from the safety of a world of endless possibilities – all of which were but a click away – back into a bleak reality of depressed, warring parents and of a felt-to-be inhospitable body that left her feeling undesirable.

The missed sessions were also expressions of what she needed to avoid in our relationship. Coming to see me was experienced in the transference as being exposed to my undesiring, and hence felt-to-be-critical glare. If ever I took up in the sessions how she shut me out, she would shrug and say, "I'm not in the mood today", but more often she simply remained silent. Sharon did, however, sometimes bring dreams and it is through her dreams that we were able, painstakingly and over time, to begin to understand the encumbrance that was her body, and the way in which cyberspace allowed her to escape from the reality of her embodied self. I would now like to illustrate this with clinical material over several weeks taken from the end of our first year of work together.

After missing two weeks of therapy because she had felt so low that she had been unable to leave the house, Sharon arrived for her session irritable. She told me that she'd had enough of therapy, that it wasn't helping and that it was, to use her words, "a waste of time". She said that talking and looking at her dreams was not giving her any practical help. Her mother had told her to ask me to give her some advice to help her to get out of bed in the morning. It had been her mother who had got her up that morning and made her come, but she had only come because she wanted to tell me that she was going to end the therapy. And yet as I listened to her I sensed that she had come because she was desperate.

I said that even though she had told me that talking and looking at her dreams had been unhelpful, I thought that she had nevertheless made the effort to come because she knew she was in trouble and wanted me to help her to stay in the therapy. She remained immobile and silent for several minutes and then, as if in trance like state, told me of the dream she had the night before:

> I am in a dark cave and can't see anything. I try to get out but my body keeps bumping into hard things and I can feel blood gushing out of my leg. I felt sick and tired and I curled up in a corner hoping I would die.

I said that she was in a lot of pain and that she wanted me to know this and help her to shed some light on what was making her feel so bad. Sharon rolled up the sleeve of her cardigan and showed me some superficial cuts, as well as a new tattoo she had done the previous week – her only excursion out of the house. She said, without affect, and as she looked at her arms, "It is painful … I guess".

I said that her body bore the marks of the pain she felt inside and that perhaps, as in her dream, she hoped that if her body died, the pain would stop. Sharon replied that she hated her body and that she had spent the last two weeks wishing she were dead. She had only managed, she said, because she played a lot of computer games and that had taken her mind "off it".

I said that coming to see me must feel like having to switch thinking back 'on' and that this felt like me asking a lot of her. Sharon replied that she thought she was beyond help. I said that being in her body felt like being trapped in a dark cave she cannot escape from. She nodded and said that she hated her body. I observed that when she played her games she could forget about her body. She nodded and said it was "like being someone else … being free … Claire [one of her avatars] is so cool … she's pretty and smart and no-one messes her about".

It was at this point that the trance-like state gave way once again to a more dismissive tone. She became fidgety and looked immediately bored: "I've had enough of talking". I felt jolted by this as if she had disconnected herself from me as suddenly as she had briefly connected. I wondered whether this disconnection had been triggered by an awareness of how much she longed for my attention and yet, in the transference, she was often relating to me as someone who would reject her so it was safest to withdraw and reject me first. Indeed, this was a pattern of exchange between us that dominated much of the therapy: brief excursions into our relationship where we could meet and think together were invariably followed by more protracted periods when she shut me out and she comforted herself with the fantasy that she did not need anyone and hence would not be hurt by anyone.

The next session was a particularly tumultuous one because her computer had broken down during the week and she had not been able to access her games for several days except on her Nintendo, which was not the same.[3] She was restless and highly irritable, impatient with my attempts to relate to her. She came across as less articulate than was usual for her; she was confused and struggling to form thoughts. I thought she had decompensated markedly in the intervening week, as if the loss of access to her virtual world had disoriented her, exposing her brutally to a real world she could barely relate to or think about.

She eventually told me that she had felt very "bored" and that she hated not having something to do with her time. I wondered with her as to whether she was feeling confused and frightened, which she called 'bored'. At this point her more dismissive façade gave way and she quickly became distressed, telling me that she had missed an interview to explore a place at a college (she had forgotten about it), and that her father had told her he would no longer support her, that she had to go out to work. She told me anxiously that she was not able to work, that she could not manage this. She then described in detail how unwell she had also been feeling, gripped by a gastric virus which had caused diarrhoea: "I was out buying some gum and I thought I was going to lose it and shit everywhere", she told me.

I said that she was letting me see just how dangerous it felt when she lost access to the only space in which she was relieved of this body that kept pulling her down: without that escape she feared that all her messy, shitty feelings would leak out everywhere. She nodded and said that it had all been made worse by waking up that morning to find her bed sheets soaked in blood.

At her worst Sharon so disregarded the reality of her body that her menstrual cycle could catch her by surprise, as it had evidently done the night before. She told me that her mother had got very upset about this and shouted at her. Her father had taken one look and told her that she "disgusted" him. As she related this she sounded fragile and humiliated and I became acutely aware of the physical, visual relationship between us. I said that she was bringing this powerful image of her blood stained sheets as proof of just how difficult it was to escape this hated body, that somehow it always inevitably left its mark, exposing her to the harsh, critical glare of others including, now, my eyes that left her fearing my judgement of her.

Sharon sat back in the chair and pinched the skin on her face: "I hate this", she said and then she pulled out of her coat pocket the Nintendo she often carried around with her. I said she had brought a lot of painful feelings today and that she was now retreating into the safe, predictable world of her games. Despite numerous attempts on my part to reach her, Sharon remained glued to her Nintendo until the end of the session. But watching her was in itself instructive: she tapped away furiously, engrossed in the activity, seemingly confident in her dexterity, and ultimately triumphant as she scored against thinking and the awkwardness of our respective physical presence in the room. I was left feeling redundant as I witnessed first hand the seduction of the certainty that the machine afforded her and that pulled her away from a real interaction with me.

It was clear that my attempt to take up the transference with her had not relieved her; rather, it seemed to turn me precisely into the kind of harsh, critical object she feared. As she shut me out I felt peculiarly exposed and became acutely aware of myself in my body and very uncomfortable in it, as if I had now become identified with her felt-to-be physically repulsive self.

The next week she returned and told me this "horrible" dream:

> I am floating ... I feel so light ... I look below and all I see are dots, moving around, close together and then they start to get bigger and bigger and they spread everywhere... it's disgusting, like some kind of gluey mess.

Sharon eventually went on to tell me that her parents had a big row and her father had hit her mother the night before and he had then left the house. She did not know if he would be back. She said she did not care one way or another. She was then silent. I said that when things got very difficult at home, and in her mind, she retreated into a safer place in her mind where she could escape from the physical reality of where she was – a 'higher' place from where big problems could seem so small, like tiny dots in the distance. And yet, as in her dream, these dots eventually grew bigger and bigger – they didn't simply go away, they left a gluey mess behind in which she felt stuck.

Unusually for her, Sharon replied immediately and more thoughtfully. She said that she hated living at home, that it was so hard to hear her parents arguing all the time and seeing her father hit her mother. She said that she had coped by putting her headphones on and playing games. When she played, she said that she felt "peaceful, safe, like I'm not on my own anymore". She then told me that she had another dream earlier in the week in which she had an accident and she was on a life support machine, with tubes doing all the work of keeping her alive. She said she could not recall anything else except that "it felt good".

When I asked for some associations to the dream Sharon said that she had heard on the radio an item about someone who had been left "like a kind of vegetable" after a motorbike had crashed into a car and that everyone was saying what a terrible thing this had been. Instead, she had thought to herself, "Lucky bastard – this is better than being alive and having to do all this stuff for yourself – at least he is fed, changed, taken care of".

I said that she had witnessed another terrible crash between her parents and this left her feeling impotent and frightened, but that she did not know how to manage these feelings in herself. She felt her only option was to make herself not feel anything, to plug herself into her 'life support' computer-machine. Sharon replied that there was "no point to feeling because there is nothing I can change".

Discussion

I will not go further into this last session. Suffice to say that these excerpts from three consecutive sessions are very representative of the first year of our work together. They illustrate the pain of thinking, the disturbing nature of being-in-a-body, and the hopelessness Sharon felt in relation to her predicament: "nothing can change". Faced with this feeling, cyberspace was a welcoming haven in which she could manipulate her world and her own self-representation at will.

For Sharon, the body was an obstacle that had to be constantly managed and triumphed over, typically through its denial and the consequent retreat into the safe cocoon provided by cyberspace – the computer and the space it linked her into became quite literally a kind of life support machine, that is, it supported Sharon in managing the demands of reality by providing an alternative to it. The images in her second dream of her "floating" and feeling "light" aptly capture the absence of a body weighing her down and rooting her in the hard reality that, by contrast, she painfully bumps into in the "dark cave" of the first dream.

The image of the life support machine is especially relevant to this discussion since it also captures another feature of cyberspace that I would like to draw attention to, namely the way in which the relationship to the computer, and the space it gives access to, parallels the wished for, pre-Oedipal relationship to a receptive, desiring maternal body that can be fully known and controlled. The computer's responsiveness could be understood as giving Sharon access to a good 'screen mother' – always there, except when it breaks down and then Sharon is once again 'dropped'. She feels enraged and then frightened, and her capacity to respond to the cues from her real body is severely undermined. In the transference, the visual relationship between us becomes central, at times leaving her feeling at the mercy of what she experienced at best as my disinterest and at worst as a more active rejection because I had a more desirable other in my mind.

Sharon evidently experienced herself as profoundly undesirable in her mother's eyes in particular, which she felt were more drawn to her brother. Her body was felt to be messy, disgusting, always leaking and exposing her to the critical eyes of the object. She tried to counter this experience by searching for an alternative, more desirable image of her body through her made-up self in a virtual world, or through her fantasies of cosmetic surgery. These simulated versions of herself allowed her to temporarily create a connection to a fantasised responsive, desiring maternal body. I want to stress, too, the relationship to the computer itself because as Sharon related it to me, and as I witnessed for myself in the session when she played with the Nintendo, the physicality of the machine and the way it almost moulded into her body – and became an extension of it – powerfully reinforced the fantasy of control/fusion with the maternal object/body with which it had become identified.

As will be clear, Sharon was a very depressed young girl who was on the edge of, or in, a psychotic state of mind much of the time. Cyberspace provided her with an extension of the psychotic space that she retreated into in her mind. In this kind of space, the reality of the real world was disavowed and the quality of Sharon's painful experience was reduced to a kind of intoxication with the virtual promise of a disembodied self and other whom she could access when she wished. When she could not access this state of mind she effectively broke down as the reality of the body violently intruded (as with her menstrual cycle soiling the sheets).

Being a no-body

Paul was just under 17 years of age when his parents sought help for him privately. They were concerned that he had become withdrawn, spending long periods of time on the Internet, using social networking sites and playing a variety of computer games. They had been very tolerant at first because they thought that he would soon tire of this, but when he did not his mother in particular started to worry.

Paul was an only child. Both his parents were very gifted academics, who devoted a great deal of time to their own research and interests. They prized independence and had adopted the stance that Paul would "learn from his mistakes", that "reason would triumph", and hence they did not keep a close eye on him. Like them, Paul was also very cerebral and schoolwork had always proved easy for him. On meeting him, however, it was clear that he inhabited his body with less ease: he seemed awkward in his movements, his choice of clothes was very conservative and lacked any personal stamp, his manner was tentative. He sat in my chair on our first meeting, perched on its edge for the whole session, without even taking his coat off on a hot summer's day.

When I asked him why he had come he replied that he did not want to worry his parents. He told me that they thought he worked too hard and did not go out enough with friends. With some difficulty he was able to tell me that he felt he was not amusing or entertaining like many of his friends were, and that he was "awkward" in social situations. He did not have a girlfriend, and he emphasised that he had no interest in having a relationship, but he chatted to a lot of girls on social networking sites. This suited him, he said, but he also added that sometimes he felt lonely – as far as I was concerned this acknowledgement was the most hopeful statement he had made in this session. He rounded off this discussion with a pithy "I'm a nobody". At this stage he did not mention the use of the Internet.

As the months passed the sessions developed a clear pattern: he came, he dutifully listened to whatever I said, and he left without making much of an impression on me such that I often found I forgot what he said or what I had said. The first important development took place around the ninth month of our work together, after he had fallen and sustained a cut requiring several stitches. His mother had left me a message to say she was deeply worried as he had stopped eating and spent all his time on the Internet.

He came for his session five days after this incident, looking very down-trodden. At first he was very silent, and then he offered this dream:

> I am walking slowly and as I walk I see a house collapsing. There is dust everywhere and I get covered in this dust. I can't breathe. I fall to the ground and cannot get back up.

He gave no associations to the dream, but after a long silence he volunteered that he was fascinated by images of detonating buildings and that he often searched the Internet for these images. He had been gripped by the collapse of the Twin Towers. He was quick to add that his interest in this event was simply in the images of the fallen buildings, reduced to dust. Since the terrorist attacks he had avoided lifts and tall buildings, he said, and he added, "Actually I have always been afraid of buildings collapsing. As a child I always read about earthquakes … they fascinate me". He then mentioned, almost in passing, that he had fallen.

I said that his fall had deeply unsettled him as if it had reminded him that he had a body and that a body was like a building: it *could* collapse or explode and be messy, but he was now not dealing with an image of someone else's body or of a building collapsing – it was *his* body. Paul looked away, evidently uncomfortable with my mention of the body, and I commented on this. Paul said that he wished he could forget the body and "have no body". He said he far preferred "being in my head". I said that his body seemed like a scary place to be in, so scary that it was preferable to be 'a no-body'. Paul smiled furtively as if he recognised my reference to what he had said in our first meeting and, I thought, felt understood.

He then proceeded to tell me for the first time that he had met a girl on one of the social networking sites he visited and with whom he had exchanged a lot of e-mails and texts. After months of virtual exchanges she had upped the ante and suggested that they should meet up. It was, interestingly, after this suggestion that he had gone for a walk – "to clear my mind", as he put it – and he had crashed into a lamppost, tripped and fallen. When he saw the blood he said that he had felt like throwing up, that it disgusted him. He said he had not felt as if it was his body that he was seeing or touching.

I said that the thought of actually meeting this girl in the flesh had been deeply troubling as if he had been forced suddenly into having to think about a real relationship – about sex – rather than a relationship he largely controlled in his mind. For the first time Paul told me that he had never kissed a girl, let alone had sex. He added that the thought of kissing actually repulsed him. All he could see was "an exchange of saliva", which disgusted him. When he had been exchanging e-mails with the girl he had told her he wanted to have sex with her, but he had not really meant this. In his fantasy he had imagined long talks with the girl, "perhaps stroking her hair", he said, but it never went beyond this.

He then recalled being a little boy and spending summers in a mountain resort with his mother while the father wrote his books. His mother would read to him and stroke his hair. He became tearful as he told me this. It was the first time he had ever shown any live feeling in the session. I said he so longed to be this little boy, sitting with his mother, enjoying being alone with her and having all of her attention. I said that it was this kind of image that he had in his mind as he communicated with this girl, but that as soon as she wanted to transpose their relationship into the real world of real bodies he became terrified.

Paul was silent and I sensed his discomfort in his body in a very direct way. In my countertransference I also became acutely aware of my own physicality. I said that I could see that as we spoke together about these things the real world of real bodies was live in the room between us and that he felt very unsettled by it, not sure how to relate to me as a woman.

I will not go further into this session but it is worth noting that where the denial of the body is central to the individual's psychic equilibrium, the sexual transference is typically avoided, and sometimes not just by the patient. It can indeed prove very difficult to take it up. Even when taken up, the interpretation can be resisted by the patient, but its eventual working through typically yields helpful developments in the therapeutic work.

Discussion

Paul's feeling that he was "a nobody" was an apt description of how the denial of the reality of his body – a no-body – was at the root of his emotional and social difficulties and his retreat into cyberspace. As the work progressed it became clearer that as a young child he had enjoyed an overly close relationship with his mother. She had seemingly felt very neglected by the husband's investment in his work and had turned to Paul for comfort. When he was 12 she had, however, resumed her career and Paul experienced this as being brutally cast aside. This expulsion coincided with the onset of puberty. This had left Paul profoundly confused about his changing body and the part it played in disrupting this more blissful pre-Oedipal union with his mother. In order to manage the internal confusion, he had to find ways of bypassing the body.

Over the Internet Paul could indulge once more in his fantasies of an uninterrupted closeness with a woman/mother. He could even write about sex without this posing a problem until he was taken at his word. Then, he literally crashes into something, trips and the sight of blood coming from his body is deeply disturbing to him. I thought that the "crashing" into the lamppost, followed by falling and the sight of blood, evoked his fantasy of sexual intercourse as a bloody exchange of fluids that disgusted him. Indeed he told me in a subsequent session that he had been very affected by one of his friends telling him about "the blood when you have sex with a virgin".

Paul's preoccupation with, and excitement about, detonating, falling buildings could be read in a number of ways, of course. His aggression and fear of the damage he could cause are evident. The buildings seemed to me to be a powerful metaphor for the maternal body – that fantasised house in which he lived tied to his mother – and which was forever threatened with collapse by the Oedipal rival, and by his own hatred and attacks on the body that he felt had so brutally expelled him. The sexual imagery conjured up by the detonated building will be apparent: it was evidently exciting to him, and yet these images (actual or in his mind) were never used to masturbate since Paul could not allow himself to masturbate. Even so, we were able over time to understand how his search for these images reflected his preoccupation with his sexual body – a body he feared and that he experienced as proof that he had lost his mother forever.

Conclusion

The delicate and intricate processes that support the establishment of a secure sense of self confidently rooted in the body, and the capacity to reflect on experience rather than enact it on, and through, the body, can be undermined by the relentless emphasis on transformation, change and triumph over the body now made possible by a staggering range of new technologies. I have suggested that these external trends do not cause new forms of psychopathology, but rather that they impinge on how we negotiate the task of integrating body and mind into a coherent image and experience of ourselves. In this chapter I have suggested that the merger of body and machine, and access to cyberspace, may impact adversely on the course of the adolescent process in some vulnerable young people, and more specifically on the young person's capacity to integrate the reality of the body into the self-representation.

Faced with the external complexity of the demands of the modern world (especially for young people), and the internal complexity and pain inherent in what is psychically required to develop a body and mind that feel one's own, it is tempting to retreat into virtual spaces where the reality of the body is either denied altogether, or where the body becomes solely an instrument for personal gratification, reassurance and comfort, not the basis for a connectedness with others. For some young people, like Sharon and Paul, immersion in virtual reality becomes psychically *necessary* in order to control an otherwise disturbing otherness that resides in the body.

Notes

1 I am using the terms cyberspace and virtual reality interchangeably.
2 For the reasons I outline I am using this term in preference to 'body image' or 'body representation', but not as distinct from these terms. The body imagining is, however, not to be equated with the body of Lacan's Imaginary.
3 This was probably on account of the fact that console games like Super Mario Bros. limit the user's control of the avatar. For example, the player cannot decide how Mario looks.

References

Abraham, K. (1924) A Short Study of the Development of the Libido Viewed in Light of Mental Disorders. In K. Abraham (1979) *Selected Papers on Psychoanalysis*. London: Maresfield.

Allison, S. von Wahide, L., Shockley, T. and Gabbard, G. (2006) The Development of the Self in the Era of the Internet and Role-Playing Fantasy Games. *American Journal of Psychiatry, 163*: 381–385.

Anzieu, D. (1990) *A Skin for Thought: Interviews with Gilbert Tarrab on Psychology and Psychoanalysis*. London: Karnac.

Arias, R., Soifer, R. and Wainer, A. (1990) Disavowal of the Danger of Nuclear War: Effect of Cultural Factors on Mental Attitudes. *The International Review of Psycho-Analysis, 17*: 89–95.

Baudrillard, J. (1988) *America*. London: Verso.

Bion, W. (1970) *Attention and Interpretation*. London: Maresfield.

Blos, P. (1967) The Second Individuation Process of Adolescence. *Psychoanalytic Study of the Child, 22*: 162–186.

Bronstein, C. (2009) Negotiating Development: Corporeal Reality and Unconscious Phantasy in Adolescence. *Bulletin of the British Psychoanalytical Society, 45*(1): 17–26.

Curtis, A.E. (2007) The Claustrum: Sequestration of Cyberspace. *Psychoanalytic Review, 94*, 99–139.

Dini, K. (2009) Internet Interaction: The Effect on Patient Lives and Analytic Process. *Journal of the American Psychoanalytic Association, 57*(4): 979–988.

Ervin, B., Turk, C., Heimberg, R., Fresco, D. and Hantula, D. (2004) The Internet: Home to a Severe Population of Individuals with Social Anxiety Disorder? *Journal of Anxiety Disorders, 18*: 629–646.

Erikson, E. (1968) *Identity*. London: Faber.

Ewald, F. (1993) Two Infinities of Risk. In B. Massumi (Ed.) *The Politics of Everyday Fear*. Minneapolis, MN: University of Minnesota Press.

Ferrari, B. (2004) *From the Eclipse of the Body to the Dawn of Thought*. London: Free Association Books.

Fenichel, O. (1945) *The Psychoanalytic Theory of Neurosis*. New York: Norton.

Flanders, S. (2009) On the Concept of Adolescent Breakdown. *Bulletin of the British Psychoanalytical Society, 45*(1): 27–34.

Fonagy, P. and Target, M. (1996). Playing With Reality: I. Theory of Mind and the Normal Development of Psychic Reality. *International Journal of Psychoanalysis, 77*: 217–233.

Foucault, M. (1980) *Power/Knowledge: Selected Interviews and Other Writings*. New York: Pantheon.

Freud, S. (1923) The Ego and the Id. *Standard Edition, 19*: 1–66.

Freud, S. (1930) Civilization and its Discontents. *Standard Edition, 21*: 59–145.

Gaddini, E. (1969) On Imitation. *International Journal of Psychoanalysis, 50*: 475–484.

Gaddini, E. (1984) Se e Come Sono Cambiati i Nostri Pazienti Fino ai Nostri Giorni. *Rivista Di Psychoanalisi, 30*: 560–580.

Gibbs, P.L. (2007) Reality in Cyberspace: Analysands' Use of the Internet and Ordinary Everyday Psychosis. *Psychoanalytic Review, 94*: 11–38.

Guignard, S. (2008) Envy in Western Society: Today and Tomorrow. In P. Roth and A. Lemma (Eds) *Envy and Gratitude Revisited*. London: Karnac.

Haag, G. (1985) La Mère et le Bébé dans les Deux Moities du Corps. *Neuropsychiatrie de l'enfance, 33*: 107–114.

Hägglund, T. and Piha, H. (1980) The Inner Space of the Body Image. *Psychoanalytic Quarterly, 49*: 256–283.

Hockney, D. (1990) Quoted in W. Leith, *Independent on Sunday*, 21 October 1990, p. 37.
Josipovici, G. (1986) *Touch*. Newhaven: Yale University Press.
Krueger, D. (1989) *Body Self and Psychological Self*. New York: Brunner/Mazel.
Krueger, D. (2004) Psychodynamic Perspectives on Body Image. In T. Cash and T. Pruzinsky (Eds) *Body Image: A Handbook of Theory, Research and Clinical Practice*. New York: Guilford.
Laufer, E. (no date) The Body as Internal Object. Unpublished conference paper.
Laufer, M. (1968) The Body Image, the Function of Masturbation and Adolescence: Problems of the Ownership of the Body. *Psychoanalytic Study of the Child, 23*: 114–137.
Laufer, M. and Laufer, E. (1984) *Adolescence and Developmental Breakdown*. New Haven, CT: Yale University Press.
Lemma, A. (2010) *Under the Skin: A Psychoanalytic Study of Body Modification*. London: Routledge.
Lichtenberg, J. (1975) The Development of the Sense of Self. *Journal of the American Psychoanalytic Association, 23*: 357–385.
Lichtenberg, J. (1978) The Testing of Reality from the Standpoint of the Body Self. *Journal of the American Psychoanalytic Association, 26*: 453–484.
Mahler, M. and Furer, M. (1968) *On Human Symbiosis and the Vicissitudes of Individuation*. New York: International Universities Press.
Meltzer, D. (1967) Identification and Socialization in Adolescents. *Contemporary Psychoanalysis, 3*: 96–103.
Morahan-Martin, J. (2008) Internet Abuse: Emerging Trends and Lingering Questions. In A. Barak (Ed.) *Psychological Aspects of Cyberspace: Theory, Research, Application*. Cambridge: Cambridge University Press.
Pratarelli, M. (2005) Sex, Shyness and Social Internet Use. Paper presented at the 114th Annual Conventions of the American Psychological Association, Washington D.C.
Raphaell-Leff, J. (forthcoming) Aliens and Alienation: Mind Invaders and Body Snatchers (under review).
Raulet, G. (1991) The New Utopia: Communication Technology. *Telos, 87*: 51.
Robins, K. and Webster, S. (1999) *Times of Techno-Culture: From the Information Society to the Virtual Life*. London: Routledge.
Rey, H. (1994) *Universals of Psychoanalysis and the Treatment of Psychotic and Borderline States*. London: Free Association Books.
Sand, S. (2007) Future Considerations: Interactive Identities and the Interactive Self. *Psychoanalytic Review,* 94: 83–97.
Sandler, J. (1994) Phantasy, Defence and the Representational World. *Infant Mental Health,* 15: 26–35.
Schilder, P. (1950) *The Image and Appearance of the Human Body*. New York: International Universities Press.
Sigman, A. (2009) Well Connected? The Biological Implications of Social Networking. *Biologist, 56*(1): 14–20.
Sjödin, C. (2006) Ill-Health in Sweden 2005: Discontent in a Modern Welfare Society and its Relation to Globalization. *International Forum of Psychoanalysis, 15*: 139–145.

Suler, J. (2002) Identity Management in Cyberspace. *Journal of Applied Psychoanalytic Studies*, *4*, 455–460.

Suler, J. (2004) Computer and Cyberspace Addiction. *Journal of Applied Psychoanalytic Studies*, *1*, 359– 362.

Suler, J. (2008) Cyber-Therapeutic Theory and Techniques. In A. Barak (Ed.) *Psychological Aspects of Cyberspace: Theory, Research, Application*. Cambridge: Cambridge University Press.

Toronto, E. (2009) Time out of Mind: Dissociation in the Virtual World. *Psychoanalytic Psychology, 2*: 117–133.

Turkle, S. (1995) *Life on the Screen: Identity in the Age of the Internet*. New York: Touchstone.

Turkle, S. (2005) *The Second Self: Computers and the Human Spirit*. Cambridge: MIT Press.

Whang, L., Lee, F. and Chang, G. (2003) Internet Overuses Psychological Profile: A Behavior Sampling Analysis of Internet Addiction. *Cyberpsychology and Behavior*, 6: 143–150.

Winnicott, D.W. (1966) Psycho-Somatic Illness in its Positive and Negative Aspects. *International Journal of Psychoanalysis, 47*: 510–516.

Winnicott, D.W. (1972) Basis for Self in the Body. *International Journal of Child Psychotherapy*, *1*: 7–16.

Woods, S. (2002) *Working with Adolescents*. London: Palgrave.

Wood, H. (2006) Compulsive Use of Internet Pornography. In J. Hillier, H. Wood and W. Bolton (Eds) *Sex, Mind and Emotion*. London: Karnac.

Yang, S. and Tung, C. (2007) Comparison of Internet Addicts and Non-Addicts in Haiwanese High School. *Computers in Human Behavior, 23*: 79–96.

Ybarra, M., Alexander, C. and Mitchell, K. (2005) Depressive Symptomatology, Use, Internet Use and On-line Interaction: A National Survey. *Journal of Adolescence Health, 36*: 9–18.

Zizek, S.L. (2004) What can Psychoanalysis Tell us About Cyberspace? *The Psychoanalytic Review, 91*: 801–830.

Chapter 6

"A perfect world" and its imperfections

Psychoanalytic clinical notes on adolescence and virtual reality

Vincenzo Bonaminio

"Is psychic space on the point of disappearing?"

"John, you are an analog alarm clock in a digital era." With these words, the "villain of the day," arrogant and self-confident, turns to Bruce Willis, the "die hard" character John McClane, the bold policeman who uses his body, strength, and good fortune to resolve impossible situations. Gradually, in the sequels to this successful film series, these impossible situations become ever more dominated by computerized and multimedia techniques.

In my opinion, this statement (banal but expressive, if you will) accurately portrays, in a graphic and concise way, the growing gap that exists between a certain manner in which an analyst presents himself, and that in which the "new patients" – and among these, children and adolescents – conduct themselves in sessions. That is, *there is a risk of the analyst being like an analog alarm clock in a digital era.*

With the expression "the new patients," I am referring to patients of the contemporary, current era (without, however, engaging in a detailed argument) – fundamentally, those patients who suffer from *disturbances of their own subjectivity*, of the *meaning of existence*, of their *sense of being* (of the "*possibility of being*," as Wright [1988] would say). They bring to analysis psychological problems of living, of lifestyle, and of psychopathology that are different from those of so-called classical patients – admittedly, if "classical patients" exist or ever existed – on whom the psychoanalytic technique was modeled and to whom we still make reference, and rightly so.

In some ways, the term "the new patients" relates to Julia Kristeva's writing. With the expression *les nouvelles maladies de l'âme* – which she used as the title of her book *New Maladies of the Soul* (1993) – this noteworthy French author emphasizes that the essential feature of the "new forms of discontent" that are arriving in the analyst's consulting room is that they are characterized by "difficulties in representation." Kristeva asks whether the psychic space, this "dark room" of our identity, where the misfortunes of living are reflected simultaneously with joy, with freedom, is on the brink of disappearing. But it is not this line of thought that I intend to develop, even though it is undoubtedly connected to my argument. I will briefly return to this later.

In this chapter I will focus, instead, on adolescents in analysis. Adolescents as our patients – and more generally adolescence as both a phase and a life condition – are deeply affected by the impact of the frantic transformations imposed upon our lives by the growing impact of virtual reality, which is already become a constituent part of our everyday life.

The question of whether "psychic space is on the point of disappearing," in my view, needs to be reformulated in the following terms: psychic space is not on the point of disappearing, but is undergoing a process of metamorphosis – one so multifaceted and fast-paced in its transformations that it could give the *false impression* that psychic space, as we analysts have described it for decades, is on the edge of disappearing.

In these times, as analysts, we need to be open-minded and not cling to old certainties. We should be able to *recognize* the invariants of *the individual living in a psychic space* and the new forms that it is assuming. Clinically, this requires that we give consideration to both invariants and new forms, in order to understand how they intermingle with each other and together form a new reality, a new clinical reality. New clinical pictures are created, but these may not be recognized as such and may be interpreted psychopathologically, according to a certain technical rationale – a frame of reference that is no longer applicable. This situation can have consequences in clinical practice more generally, in diagnostic assessments and in recommended treatment parameters (for example, frequency of sessions), which may be arrived at through misunderstandings about the quality and substance of the adolescent patient's psychopathology. Thus, one may risk falling either into the trap of *de-pathologizing* certain behavioral patterns that have become "common ways of living," or, just the opposite, falling into the trap of *hyper-pathologizing* particular clinical behaviors (such as the use of video games as a defense and a withdrawal *tout court*).

There can also be consequences that impact directly on clinical technique. For example, the analyst may be misled into deciding against an interpretation that highlights the defensive function of some ways of living in virtual space, ways that prevent a relationship with parts of the self – that glorify omnipotence, that intensify dissociation between areas of psychic experience. Or, on the other hand, the analyst might be interpretively too insistent – especially in terms of the transference – in regard to lifestyles that he, the analyst (from his old-fashioned point of view), considers defensive, narcissistically pathological, and constituting denial of "real reality," while for the patient they have a very different meaning.

In other words, we find ourselves navigating a clinical technique that has to be steered within the narrow straits of Scylla and Charybdis, one that must avoid both dangers.

Adolescence today

The vignette taken from an adolescent's psychoanalytic treatment – to which I will refer in the second part of this paper – is intended to illustrate precisely this risk: of the analyst's *unpreparedness*, that is, to grasp on a technical level the changeable nature of the clinical pictures that our new patients bring to analysis. This is neither a matter of being "modern," assuming today's reality as an inescapable fact, nor is it an act of clinging to ancient interpretive certainties.

As I state further along in my clinical example, if I had been aware of what my young patient's psychopathology foretold – that is, that over the next ten years there would be an explosion in the virtual world – I would have better understood his anxieties, I think. I would have been closer to understanding his self state, and perhaps I would have been capable of formulating more specific interpretations, and thus been of greater help to him without having to make the slightest change to the clinical methodology or technique, or to how I listened to the patient and provided him with appropriate, well-timed interpretations.

I am fully aware that this is not an easy task; our certainties are threatened. I have to admit that I too have been a victim of this urge to cling on to "classical beliefs" because I have most acutely felt the disorganizing impact of the "John McClane analyst" – the one endowed with an analog instrument in the face of the patient's digital armament – in working with adolescent patients.

As analysts we are not so much the better "judges of things" because of our supposed closeness and familiarity with the unconscious (Bonaminio, 2005). Rather, by virtue of our psychoanalytic practice, we are positioned at a peculiar intersection of what Freud (1929) called "civilization's discontents." We are not only and simply in the position to "observe" the rapid and continual social and cultural transformations with our cognitive instruments, forged on a social and cultural reality quite distinct from the present. We cannot fool ourselves into thinking we stand on the banks of a river in flood, that is, outside its maelstrom. The so-called "crisis of psychoanalysis" – about which psychoanalysts, sometimes as *laudatores temporis acti*, masochistically consult one another – stems from the crisis of thinking of ourselves as part of global society; this is itself an aspect of civilization's discontent. As Widlöcher (1996) writes, we need to have, and must have, new maps for psychoanalysis.

In dealing clinically with the "reality of the virtual reality" in which our adolescent patients live, we have to trace a new, tentative map, so to speak. This map will gradually become more accurate and more complete through clinical comparison of the work of many practicing analysts in a spirit of open inquiry that is not prejudiced *against* the new virtual reality.

I have also chosen to focus on adolescence in this chapter because I am of the view that we should regard this phase of life as our one privileged observatory, due to its function as a cultural link between generations. As Kaës (1998, p. 128) noted, "the new forms of civilization's discontents disturb the structuring and functioning of psychic life, and especially the processes of transformation and mediation, which are the most fragile and sensitive to the meta-psychic effects of intersubjectivity." As an observatory, adolescence gives us the chance to see, almost in real time, how rapid, overwhelming, transient, and "ungraspable" are the changes in ways of thinking, of representing inner and external reality – how incipient and at the same time abortive they may be. Adolescence highlights aspects of civilization's discontents, and along with these, the discontents of the analyst who has to face them (Bonaminio, 2005; 2011; in press).

Listening to adolescents' discourse allows us to focus on aspects of psychic material in terms of contemporary culture. We can observe the installation and continuing existence of trauma in the interior psychic fabric – that is to say, the impact on the ego of what is not yet representable, what falls outside its orbit, and what finds it unprepared, so to speak, to cope; but the ego is nevertheless influenced and its structure is altered. There is a consequent *undeveloped differentiation between fantasy and reality*, up to the point of their being equated – e.g., the virtual absence or reduction of the transitional area between the realms of fantasy and reality (see Freud, 1925; Winnicott, 1951, 1963).

In this context, it is important to keep in mind what we could call – speaking in terms of the changing features of psychic functioning and psychopathology – a sort of progressive legitimization of "autistic auto-sensuousness." This was originally described by Tustin (1981, 1983) in regard to autistic children and some "neurotic" patients. As Etchegoyen and Ahumada (2002) observe: "The autistic-mimetic psychic disturbances are becoming the mark of the age," whose consequences can also be seen in a diminishing tolerance of the classical setting in recent decades.

This legitimization of an "autistic auto-sensuousness" seems to be, at a different level, a common trait or a tendency that we find not only in the therapy of severely disturbed children and adolescents, but also in many other clinical adult conditions. In the latter, it seems to be related to a basic disturbance of the self, to a deeply rooted fragility of the narcissistic bases of personality; it appears to *defensively* perform the function of giving a temporary cohesion to what is fundamentally under the threat of dispersion. This is a *sophisticated defensive maneuver*, to paraphrase Winnicott (1967, p. 220).

Nowadays we take for granted the adolescent patient's basic need for privacy of the self, his very human need to preserve the inner nuclei of an *incommunicado* self (Winnicott, 1963, p. 187). Sometimes this appears in the clinical setting not as a need, but rather as a stated prerogative: a right to autistic auto-sensuousness. For example, the patient might say something like: "Don't bother me – I have a perfect right to be elsewhere with my mind, to be in my own world, outside of everything!" – this could be an adolescent-type statement. In this manner, what we are used to describing as a *psychic retreat* or an *emotional withdrawal* is not represented to the self and/or to the other (the analyst) as a need (actually, rather than being *represented,* it is "presented" without even minimal elaboration; in effect, it is "imposed"). Such a need might have a regressive tone that only expresses that it is malignant, i.e. only aimed at a "leave me alone! Don't bother me!" state. Here the adolescent's retreat/withdrawal is presented as a right, as a "legitimate way to exist," which denies both the self and the other, in effect passing itself off as a mandate. However, it may also be a plea for recognition of the self by the analyst (cf. Balint, 1968, pp. 119–156).

In these psychic configurations, there is, in my view, a sort of "ideological" stance, insofar as they are claims and not needs.[1] Such a stance is "ideological" in that it represents a *superstructure* – something that is in fact only falsely ideological, something that has been superimposed onto the structure. At times the structure itself is absent or is merely a *hole*, and the superstructure becomes the only thing existing.[2]

Nonetheless, such a stance fulfills a function and guarantees the adolescent a type of continuity of existence, something that may be difficult for us as practicing analysts to recognize – especially if the chart we are using to navigate in these territories is an old one, and the patient's attitude is considered only as a defense to be replaced by a more mature, less narcissistic one. In clinical practice, this is much in evidence when the analyst offers the patient interpretations, especially transference interpretations, that stem from the old chart's frame of reference. Such interpretations place a high value on interpersonal relatedness, contact, and representation. The patient's reaction to such an interpretation can be quite negative because he feels misunderstood or not understood at all. In my view, it is as though the "ideological" stance brought by the patient is *taken up*, via interpretation, by the analyst who ideologically – i.e. "falsely" – interprets the patient's behaviors. It is a trap that we are liable to fall into in the countertransference, and this will also influence the analyst's technique, perhaps in more subtle ways.

My reflections here arise out of the dismissive, highly aggressive reaction of a 14-year-old boy to my way of working – a reaction from which I learned a lot in terms of the necessity of changing standard clinical technique. To this extremely tall, arrogant boy, covered with piercings all over his body, I once interpreted, following an old, false chart (false in the sense of inauthentic), that he was retiring within himself, into the sensations arising from his piercing. (He had previously explained to me that he was continually having new piercings so as "to feel himself always done"). I said that he was cutting me off by concentrating on his Playstation because he wanted me to feel how and what *he* had felt when I had been unable to agree to his request to change one of his thrice-weekly analytic sessions so that he could go to a rave. As a consequence, he had missed the session and gone to the rave.

When I told the patient that perhaps he felt cut off by me because I had not accepted his request based on my actually not wanting him to go to the rave, and perhaps he felt that I had falsely told him I was unable to change the session, he replied quite aggressively. He used a vernacular Roman dialect, even though he came from an upper-class family and had up until then used sophisticated language:

"What the hell are you talking about – what fucked-up things are you saying? This makes no fucking sense to me! What are you talking about?"

On reflection, I understood the patient's response as a reaction to an interpretation that came from an internal position that might have been appropriate for a more "classical" patient – a less disturbed and more "structured" adolescent – but one that was not attuned to this young man's way of being and feeling. Had I interpreted not the Oedipal sense of exclusion and the "father's retaliation" for his not having complied with "the law," he might have reacted differently; for example, I might have said that I understood he was "running on empty" in terms of his psychic energy level, leading to his minimal functioning, and that he might well have needed to recharge his batteries by immersing himself in a "milky" sound that totally surrounded and pervaded him. (In fact the patient used these words to describe the experience of the rave [cf. Bonaminio, in press].) Had I taken this tack, perhaps the patient would have felt better understood via a language and a perspective nearer to his own experience. I should have seen him then more as an autistic-like boy than as a "psychologically grown-up" individual (albeit a highly disorganized and confused one).

As psychoanalysts, we are accustomed to attributing a relative stability, cohesion, and durability to those "cultural objects" (Bollas, 1992) that populate the "intermediate area" described by Winnicott – that between the individual and the social, and between the internal and external worlds. In every phase of life, cultural objects are present, not as an accessory function for psychic development, but as a fundamental nexus point, a synthesis of the *created-found* (to use Winnicott's term). These cultural objects allow a two-way osmosis between outer and inner, and provide the individual with the capacity to "sustain himself" by guaranteeing a certain stability to the confines of the self – or, we might say, to his sense of subjectivity – insofar as cultural objects are capable of incessantly transforming the self by widening its confines through *experiencing* (Bollas, 1992).[3]

Adolescence may have suffered and may be suffering from profound transformations during the present period (we could say these are infinitely more striking in the last 30 years than what may have occurred even in the relatively recent past). We analysts are like the character of the White Rabbit in *Alice in Wonderland*, who always has a watch in his hands – an analog one – and who, while muttering, "*Oh dear! Oh dear! I shall be too late!*" chases something unknown. We, too, sometimes "chase" our patients in the attempt to understand something that is beyond us, that falls outside our mentality.

We are ourselves beneficiaries of the same electronic and Internet tools that our patients use, and thus we are members of the same virtual reality that, together with them, we share (cf., Gabbard, this edition) with every other citizen of the contemporary world. For example, between sessions we send and receive e-mail; we quickly search for a particular bit of information on Google; we explore in detail on Google Earth the contours of a geographical promontory where we are going on vacation next weekend. Nevertheless, we may feel a disquieting sense of alienation from the adolescent who enters the consulting room, sits in front of us or lies down on the couch, and speaks to us almost without a break of a reality with little that is "representational," even though it apparently bears some resemblances to such. The adolescent patient tells us that he was "chatting" up to that moment with someone in one of the "communities" of which he is a member, but that someone is, or could be, only "a profile," perhaps even an intentionally changed one. The patient made an appointment for a game online; he "acquired" land on *Second Life* to "invest in an upcoming virtual building construction"; he checked his mail on *Facebook*. He read the "morning reflection" or the "evening" one – and perhaps commented on them – of the profile with the nickname "Fringuello" (whom he may not have met and may never meet). He does not know if Fringuello is male or female, what his/her age or place of residence may be, if he/she works and has a family. It is not specified that this information is included in Fringuello's profile, or in any case it could have been falsified. Discovering, perhaps, in the profile that today is the birthday of "that profile" (can one use the word *person* in this case?), and supposing that it is a woman, he may even have sent her a bouquet of flowers or some chocolates (virtual ones, of course).

A 30-year-old (but "interminably adolescent") patient told me recently that he felt very bad because "that creep of a girl whom he *didn't even know*" had "pissed him off" by not responding to his "kind thought," his "gift" – imagine that she hadn't even thanked him for the things he sent her or the witty card! Such may be the fate of "relationships" formed in cyberspace.

Nevertheless, the adolescent patient "knows" many things about this profile; he knows their secret thoughts (not necessarily authentic ones). He has a *sensual knowledge* of the profile, even though this knowledge *excludes the senses* (cf. Lemma, this edition). The adolescent patient speaks to us about that profile in his narration of the day, perhaps because he has just interrupted his chat with him, or with many others simultaneously – and that profile is thus an "object" whom he causes us to know (to paraphrase Bollas). That profile is an object that the patient "introduces" to the analyst through his narration and his free association, transporting the analyst to that place where he, the patient, met the object. The profile is an object on which to *project* something and from which to *introject* something, but that configures itself in our eyes – apparently – as a representation, even though it is not that for the patient who "presents" it.[4] And how does one regard a dream, an account of a dreamlike sequence? At times it is like this, but I have the impression that considering such material in the same way as dreams may sometimes be a defensive maneuver on the analyst's part in order to give sense to a *current reality* in that moment *inside the adolescent*. But already, *inside* is a place; it belongs to a Euclidean/Cartesian topology that has nothing to do with the continuing experience that is pervasive in the adolescent in that moment. I will return to this point later.

One could say that it is a "neo-reality" of which we know little. When I say "we know little," I am not referring to the fact that we aren't familiar with it, because in reality we are very familiar with it, more or less, because we ourselves are part of this neo-reality, this *virtual reality.* Conversely, I mean that "we don't yet know enough" – that is, enough to modify our analytic tools to include it (cf. Moreno, 2002).

To elaborate: on the one hand, so as not to exorcise it in a conservative way, we might say, "We're dealing with a flight from 'true reality,' from 'relational reality'; it is a 'narcissistic defense,' 'manic,' and must be treated as such." But does "true reality" exist? We analysts will certainly not be the ones to assert this!

Or, on the other hand, we might *passively accept it* as factual data of the modern world (or better still, the post-modern one), about which we can say nothing if we don't recognize its unavoidable and essential nature. Because of this presumed unavoidability, we may not even try to understand the psychopathological implications, those that we might alternatively, and legitimately, call the "new psychopathologies."

The diffusion of identity in a two-dimensional space

When one type of acculturation, largely linked to the family circle and written culture, is discarded in favor of an acculturation based on audiovisual media (Ahumada, 1998) that create the illusion of reality (but in reality do no more than allude to it), an "unprepared thought" is left with the arduous, traumatizing task of stabilizing the connections that appear to be inherent in this new acculturation, but that in fact are just not there, by definition. Under these new social conditions, cultural objects will be called upon all the more frequently and urgently, pressed to be "out there" mediating between the internal and the external – which of course they are powerless to do. Unconfined, the internal and external migrate from one to the other; transitional space tends to become only a tenuous membrane that contains and divides.

"Psyche is extended; knows nothing about it."[5] Freud's enigmatic statement – written in the form of incomplete jottings, only a few days before his death – can of course be interpreted in different ways. To me it appears to effectively and disquietingly prefigure the diffusion of identity, its "wanderings" in a largely two-dimensional, flat "place": the virtual world.

The pervasive impact of the social upon psychopathology comes as no news for psychoanalysis. Furthermore, as Ahumada (1998) observes, in a global society, the passing from a culture based on writing to another based on the virtual is fundamental, "because it probably represents the most shocking {e.g., traumatic} experiences on a world-wide scale to which the human species has been subjected." The possibility of *living in substitutive neo-realities and then assimilating oneself into them* emphasizes and broadens the individual's mimetic defenses in society (see Gaddini, 1984).

The "prescient" analysand and the "unprepared" analyst

My work with Ernesto, a boy who began analysis with me at the age of 11, provides a good example of how much things have changed in the past 30 years. As I have been suggesting, they have changed both internally and externally for analysts, and both internally and externally in our relationships with analysands.

Ernesto was referred to me for help with a series of typical symptoms: highly obsessive behavior, shyness, social insecurity, and a tendency to retreat from interaction with schoolmates. Furthermore, he was on the edge of dropping out of school, which shortly afterward actually happened.

Ernesto was the only child in an upper-class family. His father was a civil servant in a very high government position, and his mother, younger than her 49-year-old husband by nearly ten years, came from a "noble" southern family; she had graduated from college but did not work outside the home. Ernesto was tyrannical towards his parents, who during the assessment sessions appeared to be completely at his beck and call. They lived with the threat of his "temper tantrums that arose in response to nothing." The most relevant clinical symptom – which I came to know shortly after the first assessment session – was compulsive masturbation and the associated obsessive need to clean his hands; this had been present since he experienced premature puberty at about the age of eight. These were the basic clinical features of this early adolescent's severe psychopathology – useful for the reader, I hope, to contextualize the case.

At that time, about 30 years ago, I would have considered Ernesto to be a child in the final phase of latency and on the threshold of adolescence. Today, the definition proposed by Gutton in *Le pubertaire* (2003), "the one undergoing puberty," would be perfectly adapted to him.

Early on in the therapy, after a handful of sessions, Ernesto revealed his secret to me – a "secret" that was not really a secret; it had even been concealed by his parents in the first assessment sessions. If I had more quickly grasped the relationship between this "secret" and Ernesto's severe obsessive-compulsive behavior, that is, how his behavior served to protect the content of the secret and allowed it to live – I would certainly have assumed a different attitude in tackling the treatment of this highly intelligent, rather sly young boy.

If I had understood 30 years ago what this young boy was anticipating with his symptom, I would certainly have used a slightly different therapeutic technique. I would have taken more seriously, so to speak, his uncontrollable desire to *concretely (but virtually)* enter the world of animated cartoons, to participate in their life, to be one of them. This was Ernesto's' secret desire: he wanted to *transform himself into a small, thin figure* in order to access that world that was only apparently two-dimensional. Transformation into a small figure, he said, was the "key to entry," the only way to enter that world. (Notice here the anticipation of the "double universe," as in the 1999 film *Matrix*: the digital and the real.) Once there, he would become like them, exactly like them; he would become one of their characters, participating in their adventures and thereby modifying those exploits. (Already there were episodes that he knew by heart and for which he had imagined different developments – we might say an alternative script – because of inconsistencies he had discovered.) He would be "placed together with the cutest girl"; they would take romantic walks, play sports, and go shopping together. They would caress each other and maybe, afterward, they would make love as he had glimpsed in a suggestive scene from his favorite cartoon, "Jeeg Robot." (We are here straddling the end of the 1970s and the beginning of the '80s; nowadays that scene would be much more explicit.) But he had understood the scene and "wanted to really do that, to make love with that girl, who was his true love, *but without flesh, without sweat, without a body.*"

If only I could have understood from afar – perhaps by traveling into the future a little in my imagination – what Ernesto was anticipating with this well-developed fantasy, I would have treated him differently. I would have "cleansed" him, so to speak, of all that delirious raving that I internally attributed to him. Maybe my interpretations would have been less based on a formulation of "flight due to fear of not being able to maintain social contact with his friends." They would have been less grounded in his need to re-create a regressive set-up "where only he and Vincenzo, the analyst, could exist in *a perfect world.*" I would not have focused so much on the personality traits of the cartoon character Jeeg Robot – who was really nothing other than a normal boy, Hiroshi, whose father, Professor Shiba, was dying. The father, mortally attacked by terrible "Haniwa" soldiers, had, with one of his inventions, assigned to his son the power to transform himself into a gigantic robot, reuniting scattered parts and components in various places throughout the world – which, once they were consolidated and reassembled, gave him invincible strength. That image was highly significant in describing the patient's fear of falling to pieces and his omnipotent fantasy of reconstructing himself on a grand scale, invincible, in order to "cope with his parents' madness," which he had witnessed many times (Winnicott, 1969; Bonaminio & Di Renzo, 2008).

Perhaps I would have interpreted all this in the same way, but given less emphasis to the defensive and omnipotent aspect, and *recognized a certain plausibility* in Ernesto's desire, in his attraction to *living in a virtual world*, one less complicated, with well-established codes (which are essential in the present-day virtual world). I would have understood better and earlier the patient's need of his own self, as distorted as it might be, not only as a defense of his ego.

I would have, if I had known, but I didn't know. How could I have imagined what today is normal: treating an adolescent who says "excuse me" (if he is polite enough) when, while he is recounting a dream, he simultaneously confirms an appointment with a girl or with his friends by clicking the iPhone that is always in his hands?

Technology does matter and changes the world, including the inner one, because when Ernesto began to develop this uncontrollable wish to enter the world of animated cartoons – to be Jeeg Robot's friend, to help him, to share his exploits and perhaps also his girlfriend – his fantasy was already being sustained in part by the technological developments that were then in the early stages.

It was the time of the appearance of domestic video-registration equipment on the market, with the giant Japanese cartels led by Sony and Matsushita, which established their systems of video home entertainment in our own homes.[6]

With his tyrannical behavior, Ernesto had succeeded in getting his father to buy a sophisticated V2000 (as compensation, as we will see shortly), which had a "reverse play" feature, something other systems of the time lacked. This gave him the possibility, then, of watching and re-watching the scenes that most interested him, to the point of learning them by heart – in addition, of course, to preserving all the episodes. Ernesto could thereby also "overcome time, and no longer be a slave to it," as he somewhat surprisingly told me in a session, because while the recording was taking place, he could come to his session with me, then go home and comfortably watch his episode as many times as he liked. He said: "I'm stronger than my friends; I don't need them because I'm two Ernestos at the same time – the one who is here and the one who is recording a Jeeg Robot episode."

My interpretation of the patient's typical omnipotent fantasy of controlling all that happened was already at that time, without my being aware of it, a somewhat blunted weapon, because both of us were about to enter the digital era that before long would explode. In contrast, in speaking to him, I was still using an analog alarm clock.

What I am referring to here is not a "practical" change in technique in the sense of being less interpretive or more "tolerant" of his retreats, or of being less "psychopathologically biased" (for example, by considering his attitude less defensively omnipotent). Instead, I am questioning my capacity to be closer to the patient's experience and his need of living in a two-dimensional space; I am not thinking of his experience as merely a delusional way of escaping from the harshness of three-dimensional reality. Rather, I see it as a way of allowing his traumatized self to survive and possibly to grow. I would perhaps have interpreted this.

In the case of Ernesto, I would not want to undervalue – there at the dawning of virtual reality, but also in the virtual era itself – an *extension of time and space*, which is a different solution, different as a response to a *traumatic reality*. I have already written on this aspect of the topic, and in the interest of brevity, I refer the reader to that work (Bonaminio, 2007, 2012 in press). Here I would like to emphasize, clinically, the traumatic origin that lay at the base of Ernesto's behavior. In a manner of speaking, Ernesto was a pioneer, a forerunner of virtual reality. I will add here some clinical data about his case.

The boy was referred to me by a senior colleague who had treated his parents during a phase of acute marital disagreement – a recurrence of other, earlier periods in the couple's tormented relationship – because Ernesto, their long-awaited only child, had progressively become more insistent about refusing to attend school.

After the very early phases of the analysis, it appeared clear, reconstructively, that the young boy had knowingly used a "strategy" that appeared to be well crafted. He had first complained of physical illnesses and minor social discomforts with his schoolmates, to lower his parents' defenses and reduce their objections. They very much hoped he would perform excellently at school, but because of his complaints they tolerated his temporary refusal and intermittent attendance. Then the period of overall absence became longer, such that his eventual re-entry at school would have required a specific request at a bureaucratic level, as well as the make-up of substantial sections of the curriculum that he had missed.

At that point, Ernesto could openly declare his wish never to go back to school, to withdraw into "his world," that of animated cartoons, to end the few friendships he had (which had been – or had seemed – important until that moment). The boy's stubbornness and negativism went hand in hand with his obsessiveness, which – present all his life as a characteristic behavioral trait – at that time had a sudden, strong upsurge, such that he was hounded by the powerful need to perform obsessive rituals and by his compulsive and tormented thoughts.

With this clinical picture, the boy arrived in my office with the recommendation for an analysis, and our four sessions per week were practically the only occasion he had to leave his home – and, surprisingly, he came not unwillingly. Even then, in facing this complex clinical picture and its significant array of symptoms, I had the impression of dealing with a massive, sophisticated defense against an adolescent breakdown (Laufer & Laufer, 1984). I felt that the avoidance of an adolescent collapse and of the concrete risk of psychosis had come with a high price tag in psychic terms: the progressive impoverishment of Ernesto's emotional activity and vitality, and augmentation of his obsessive armament and of his tyrannical behavior.

I will describe only a few further aspects that are particularly significant among the various ones that I could provide to give a more complete picture of the patient's psychopathological organization and the course of his analysis. Since my purpose is to highlight this boy's "forerunner" characteristic and the analyst's relative "unpreparedness" for a new mentality that Ernesto was in fact anticipating, I cannot be other than selective in summarizing the clinical material, by focusing my attention, as mentioned, on a traumatic aspect that I believe to be of central importance.

After a "loose" and apparently fluid initiation of the analysis, Ernesto's obsessiveness was immediately conveyed, from the first sessions in the consulting room. So pronounced was his obsessiveness in organizing and dispositioning the various characters involved (little soldiers, horses, other animals, Indian tents, and little stockades of cowboys that the boy had begun to "import" from home) that the entire time of the session often passed without Ernesto being able to grant himself the luxury of "playing" – an activity that, to draw on Winnicott's remarks, was strongly desired but just as strongly precluded and prohibited, precisely as a consequence of his creativity and unpredictability.

The other element of the clinical picture that cannot be omitted was the patient's compulsive masturbation due to a difficult-to-treat genital impulse (which I will explain shortly) that could not be separated, however, from his obsessional behaviour. This was so because the boy had to recommence the masturbatory act from the start (for which he first established a rigid sequence – for example, four times) if an unpleasant thought interfered or crossed his mind. Exhausted, he would have to start the entire sequence again until he could arrive, worn out, at ejaculation, which in turn dictated an ever-increasing number of hand-washings (after execution of the masturbation itself, but also over the course of the day), such that he had developed a rather serious irritation and exfoliation of the skin of his hands.

I must add another important "historical" element before coming to the heart of the matter. The patient's compulsive masturbation, stemming from an uncontainable genital impulse, was generated and developed following his insurgent, precocious puberty at the age of eight and a half. His physical appearance (as mentioned, he was 11 when analysis began) had deceived the analyst as well; the traumatic event of early puberty had rammed into him, one might say. Slender, delicate, and rather short, Ernesto nevertheless already showed signs of a beard on his face, and the bare arms that extended from his T-shirt had an adult fuzz unusual for a preadolescent. His overall countenance, too, as well as his somewhat baritone voice, was unusual for a boy of his age.

It was Ernesto himself who told me, in a more advanced phase of the analysis – once a certain confidence and faith had gradually developed, the working alliance having been strengthened – that "*down there* [meaning his genitals] it's already like a big man's." He said that he had known and seen things that neither his parents nor anyone else imagined, and because of this he felt special and important. But he also felt like a kind of monster, a Quasimodo in an impossible search for Esmeralda. Consequently, he lived shut up in his home, as though in a tower of Notre Dame; at least there he was free to have his own thoughts and fantasies.

To complete the picture, I will describe in some detail one other aspect of the case: a "traumatic episode" that seemed to be, at least in the boy's unconscious fantasy, the origin of his precocious adolescence. Of course, it is always risky, as well as scientifically and clinically inappropriate, to make connections of a psychosomatic type to an event like precocious puberty, which is induced by a multiplicity of uncontrollable factors, neuroendocrine as well as psychic. Nevertheless, in pursuing a metaphorical line, as opposed to one of etiopathogenetic concreteness, the correlation that Ernesto made between the episode I will describe and his "having become like a big man *down there*" – and having had his first ejaculation following a strange wish to touch himself "because it felt hard" – one cannot deny that this episode has a certain dramatic, almost cinemagraphic, Fellini-esque tone. It was like a clear, lucid, sequential memory – scene after scene and frame after frame.

The episode begins with Ernesto's parents quarreling violently, even more frantically than usual. Ernesto listens to the fighting from his room, turning up the volume of the television on which he is watching his favorite cartoons. The altercation between his parents is suddenly interrupted. Two or three minutes of silence follow, in which (according to his later memory) he fears finding his mother in a pool of blood, stabbed by his father. An instant later his mother bursts into the room, telling him, "Get dressed – let's take your things and go away from here, you and I, get away from this house of hell. We'll go to Grandpa's house in Campania – he certainly loves me, and he loves you, too."

Meanwhile, Ernesto's father leaves the house – slamming the door, seized by an attack of rage. An hour or two later, the boy finds himself in a taxi with his mother, headed toward the central train station in Rome. Then they are at the track, waiting for the train. The boy has a small suitcase that his mother prepared in a rush; next to her is a porter who transports two larger bags along the platform.

The train arrives and they are about to get on, but just at that moment Ernesto's father runs up to them, panting and out of breath (he is rather overweight). Ernesto remembers his father shouting at his mother, ordering her not to leave, not to "take away *my* son!" She replies calmly and artfully, to ensure her successful escape: "I want to stay with my parents for a month or two. You can't refuse me this – it's not against the law." (Ernesto's father is a magistrate, and the boy remembers that he would never have expected his father to be involved in such a row, given the position he held.)

Mother and son spend a very tranquil period, lovingly cared for by the mother's father. The mother visits long-time friends and re-establishes contact with old high school and college companions. In the wake of his mother, Ernesto forms new friendships with the children of his mother's friends, and also explores new contacts independently of her.

It is the evening, however, that becomes the relevant moment: Ernesto's mother calls him to her side; now he is *her missing husband – she cannot be alone in bed*. The long cuddling sessions have a striking effect on Ernesto, who isn't used to such treatment. He is seduced by them, with the result that he fantasizes he really *is* his mother's husband. His genital maturity demonstrates this.

Ernesto's father makes continual and repetitive attempts to reunite the family, and finally Ernesto and his mother return to the family home at the end of the summer. It is from that moment that Ernesto begins to develop his pattern of withdrawal, obsessiveness, masturbation, and the recurrent and insistent fantasy of entering the world of animated cartoons – a fantasy that, from that time onward, seems almost frenzied to me, and against which I tend to defend myself by clinging to established technique. Jeeg Robot, who puts pieces back together to re-create a fragmented but omnipotent body, encapsulates the patient's fantasy of recomposing the "familial body" that has gone to pieces – of *transforming* it into something he knows the secret mechanisms of, that he can use to bring about a metamorphosis that will transport him from the *real world* (an intolerable one) to the virtual world (in the process of being created). The patient's "blackmail" of his father by making him buy what was then a very expensive VCR in exchange for his re-entry into the family – and as a way to attend psychotherapy sessions without missing any of his favorite episodes – seems to be, with hindsight, another way through which Ernesto can achieve Oedipal triumph over his father, devaluing him.

In looking back at the evolution of this case, I can say, like Winnicott, that I am impressed by the amount of psychic change that I personally impeded by not having known how to catch, "at the right moment," this aspect of world transformation that was taking place at that moment in the narrow, restricted space of a consulting room.

But who could have known it?

Translation by Gina Atkinson

Notes

1 Here I use the word "ideological" in the sense in which Karl Marx (in the *Grundrisse*, 1857–58) used it (which is, I think an earlier version of the concept of *false self* or *false identifications* that Winnicott [1960] later wrote about).

2 Marx writings exposed this falsified, whitewashed aspect of the exploitation of workers by capitalists; I find it an interesting theme because it is applicable to many clinical realities – whether of an individual, a group, marital couple, family, or society itself.

3 Elsewhere, I have examined in greater detail the role of "cultural objects" and "ideological objects" in adolescent development (Bonaminio, 2001).

4 Here I am intentionally using relevant terms in the sense of their original Freudian roots: *Stellung* e *Vorstellung* – "presentation," i.e., the thing in itself, essentially visual, and the representational re-cathexis of memory traces that is characteristic of the psychic work.

5 This sentence is drawn from the following passage (Freud 1941): "Space may be the projection of the extension of the psychical apparatus. No other derivation is probable. Instead of Kant's a priori determinants of our psychical apparatus. Psyche is extended; knows nothing about it."

6 At that time, at least in Italy, only the more affluent families could allow themselves to buy a VCR, which was truly a rarity and a status symbol. Or, VCRs were sometimes bought by families who weren't affluent, but had a parent who was a sort of "neo-daddy," and so with a certain level of sacrifice acquired the portable version of the VCR that included an enormous telecamera. This was used to document the son's or daughter's growth, step by step, in every possible situation of domestic life. The pile of videocassettes that preserved the child's growth, year by year, in long hours of filming, was another of the forms in which virtual reality was gradually being constructed.

References

Ahumada, J. (1998). *The Logic of the Mind*. London: Karnac.

Bollas, C. (1992). Generational awareness. In *Being a Character: Psychoanalysis and Self Experience*. New York: Farrar, Strauss & Giroux.

Bonaminio, V. (2001). Il cambiamento della nozione di spazio interno come processo introiettivo alla fine dell'adolescenza. In A.M. Nicolò (Ed.) *Adolescenza Terminata ed Interminabile*. Milano: Angeli.

Bonaminio, V. (2005). Il discorso dell'adolescente in analisi e la lacerazione del tessuto transizionale.nuove forme del disagio della civiltà. *Psiche. Rivista di cultura psicoanalitica*, *13*(2): 139–145.

Bonaminio, V. (2012). The adolescent discourse: New forms of civilizations discontents. [Modified enlarged new version of Bonaminio, V. 2005] *Psychoanal Q*. (in press).

Etchegoyen, R.H. & Ahumada, J.L. (2002). Que faire? Le rôle de la psychanalyse dans la posmodernité. In C. Botella (Ed.) *Penser les Limites. Esssais en l'honneur d'André Green*. Paris: Delachaux et Niestlé.

Freud, S. (1925). Inhibitions, symptoms and anxiety. *Standard Edition, 20*: 77–174.

Freud, S. (1941). Findings, ideas, problems. *Standard Edition*, 23: 299–300.

Gabbard, G.O. (2001) Cyberpassion: E-rotic transference on the Internet. *Psychoanal Q*, *70*: 719–737.

Gaddini, E. (1984). Changes in psychoanalytic patients up to the present day. In R.S Wallerstein (Ed.) *Changes in Analysts and Their Training*. London: IPA (Monograph 4).

Gutton, P. (2003). *Le Pubertaire*. Paris: Presses Universitaires de France.

Kaës, R. (1998). Il disagio nel mondo moderno e taluni disturbi della vita psichica: Caos nell'identità, difetti di simbolizzazione, illusione della fine delle illusioni. *Psiche, 1*(VI):122–130.

Kristeva, J. (1993). *New Maladies of the Soul*, trans. R. Guberman. New York: Columbia University Press.
Marx, K. (1857–58/2005). *Grundrisse, Foundations of the Critique of Political Economy*. London: Adult Penguin.
Moreno, J. (2002). *Ser Humano: La Inconsistencia, los Vinculos, la Crianza*. Buenos Aires: Libros de Zorzal.
Tustin, F. (1981). *Autistic States in Children*. London: Routledge/Kegan Paul.
Tustin, F. (1983). *Autistic Barriers in Neurotic Patients*. New Haven, CT/London: Yale University Press.
Widlöcher, D. (1996). *Les Nouvelles Cartes de la Psychanalyse*. Paris: Éditions Odile Jacobs.
Winnicott, D.W. (1951). Transitional object and transitional phenomena. In *Collected Papers: Through Pediatrics to Psychoanalysis*. London: Tavistock Publications.
Winnicott, D.W. (1963). Fear of breakdown. In C. Winnicott, R. Shepherd, M. Davis (Eds.) *Psychoanalytic Explorations*. London: Karnac.
Winnicott, D.W. (1967). The ætiology of infantile schizophrenia in terms of adaptive failure. In R. Shepherd, J. Jones, T. Robinson (Eds.) *Thinking about Children*. London: Karnac.
Wright, K. (1988). The possibility of being. Paper (unpublished) presented at Annual Meeting of the iW- Istituto Winnicott, Corso di psicoterapia psicoanalitica del bambino, dell'adolescente e della coppia: Integretation, Non-integration, Disintegration, Sapienza, University of Rome, 20–21 June, 2008.

Chapter 7

Internet offenders from a sense of guilt

Heather Wood

In his 1916 paper on 'Some character types met with in psycho-analytic work', Freud famously refers to 'Criminals from a sense of guilt'. He describes reports by patients of forbidden acts, committed in youth, which were done principally because they were forbidden, and which brought a sense of relief: 'Paradoxical as it may sound, I must maintain that the sense of guilt was present before the misdeed, that it did not arise from it but conversely – the misdeed arose from the sense of guilt' (p. 332). Nearly 100 years on, Freud's observation has a fresh relevance to the crime of downloading child pornography, which, in some cases, seems to be driven not primarily by sexual desire, but more in response to a persecutory internal object and the associated, primitive, sense of guilt.

There are some people compulsively using Internet pornography, and in some cases who have used and been convicted of possession of illegal (child) pornography, where the content of the images viewed, as reported in therapy, may not be overtly sadomasochistic even though the images may symbolise or imply a sadomasochistic relationship. However, these patients describe a relationship to the Internet, and the compulsion to do something 'wrong' and transgressive through the medium of the Internet, which is infused with sadomasochism.

Illegal pornography, condemned by society, provides a ready vehicle for acts of defiance against an internal object. It is as though the person communicates to this internal object, 'You think I'm bad? I'll show you "bad"'. Viewing child pornography is then not the 'best', most desirable thing they can imagine, but actually the 'worst', most despicable thing that they can think to do. This is not primarily an act of desire (though sexual gratification may be a component of it), but an act of defiance, defiance against a society perceived to be hostile and condemnatory, defiance against internal parental objects, defiance against a persecutory superego.

The crime of accessing child pornography on the Internet is a new phenomenon; the legal framework for Internet crimes was not established in England and Wales until 1998. Middleton et al. (2009) reported that Internet-related sexual offences accounted for almost a third of all sexual convictions in

England and Wales by 2005. Online sexual offending has become a major source of concern: children are exploited if not abused in the production of such images; the prevalence of this problem provides a challenge for the Criminal Justice System; there is concern about whether Internet offenders are more likely to proceed to commit a contact offence against a child; and many offenders have no prior criminal record and a proportion have had extremely responsible, sometimes high-profile public roles, suggesting that people may be drawn to act in an uncharacteristic way in their online behaviour. The apparent prevalence of an interest in paedophilic images may also be very disturbing in Western societies, which have in recent years promoted a 'zero tolerance' approach to child sexual abuse. From a clinical perspective, there is a growing demand to treat people who are anxious about their own online behaviour, those who are viewing illegal pornography and frightened of being caught, those who are alarmed by what they are drawn to view, and those who have been convicted and suffer the manifold consequences of being found guilty of an Internet child sex crime.

The popular view of such crimes is that they are manifestations of paedophilia, and that paedophilia is, in effect, akin to a sexual orientation, consisting of the sexual desire for a child. The person charged with possession of child pornography is assumed to be a longstanding paedophile, who may only have been apprehended at this point because his Internet activities have enabled him to be traced by the criminal justice system. Both of these assumptions – that the use of child pornography is driven by a primary sexual interest in children, and that paedophilia is a manifestation of sexual desire or libido – may be unwarranted. Clinical experience and the small amount of research so far available suggest that the conscious and unconscious drivers for viewing and downloading child pornography are many and varied. Child pornography may be used by those with longstanding paedophilic sexual interests in an attempt to contain existing paedophilic impulses, by providing an outlet for fantasies that are perceived to be less damaging than committing a contact offence, or it may be used to elaborate and amplify paedophilic interests. However, there are some people, perhaps those with a more obsessional profile or an autistic spectrum disorder, for whom collecting and ordering vast numbers of images comes to outweigh any overtly sexual motive; for others the quasi-social contact can be a secondary, if not a primary motive for such exchanges, particularly in those who struggle with face-to-face adult relationships. Taylor and Quayle (2003) report one of the earliest empirical studies relating to the use of Internet pornography, in which they conducted a qualitative analysis of interviews with 13 men convicted of downloading child pornography. The authors identified six discourses that served as motives for the behaviour. While sexual arousal was a key theme, sorting and collecting images was central for some, and the avoidance of real-life stresses and the facilitation of social relationships were very significant for others. As one patient said to me, 'I can't understand why, but the urge to look at pictures anaesthetises me, comforts me. Sex is only about third on the list.'

Even when sexual gratification is present, a contemporary psychoanalytic perspective would view perverse behaviours such as the viewing of child pornography as evidence of the libidinalisation of aggression, rather than an expression of libido *per se*. Freud's (1905) early view of perversions as reflecting a piece of pre-genital, infantile sexuality – that is, a manifestation of libido that has escaped repression – is well-known. Gillespie (1956) suggests that by 1910, in his paper on Leonardo, Freud had already revised this view and recognised the defensive function of perversions, and this was clearly stated in 'A child is being beaten' in 1919, and his 1927 paper on 'Fetishism'. In Freud's account of fetishism he describes how the young boy, confronted by awareness of the mother's genital and her lack of a penis, experiences acute anxiety. To fully recognise the mother's 'castration' confronts him with the possibility that he, too, might risk castration. He therefore retreats from this awareness, and invests in whatever it was that was glimpsed just before this revelation: underwear, shoes or materials such as fur, which stand for the pubic hair, for example. The fetishistic object that becomes the object of desire can then be controlled at will; it allows regression, which effectively serves to deny awareness of the mother's 'castration'; the fetish thus allows a relationship to the mother to be preserved that does not arouse unbearable anxiety. While the origin of a fetish may not occur in quite the concrete way that Freud describes, Freud recognised the function of a fetish to deny reality, to defend against castration anxiety and to reverse an experience of vulnerability, replacing this with a sense of excitement and control.

It remained for subsequent theorists, notably Payne (1939), Gillespie (1940), Glover (1933), Stoller (1975) and Glasser (1979), to recognise the primacy of aggressive rather than libidinal currents in the formation of perversions. Stoller (1975), for example, described how behaviours regarded as perverse, such as cross-dressing, can represent an act of revenge against objects felt to have attacked or denigrated the developing child's gender identity or sexuality. Through the cross-dressing ritual, Stoller suggests, the man appears to re-enact what was done to him in childhood, but at the end of the ritual, he masturbates and ejaculates, re-asserting his masculinity. Through sexualisation, the imposition of a feminine identity that was originally experienced as a trauma is transformed into an experience of triumph over the internal objects, and what was originally an experience of passive suffering, becomes an act of revenge. For Stoller, perversion is 'the erotic form of hatred', a sexualised form of aggression, and not an expression of libido *per se*.

Glasser (1979) arrived at a similar conclusion, suggesting that perversions reflect a sadomasochistic solution to claustro-agoraphobic conflicts experienced in relation to the primary object. For Glasser, separation from the primary object arouses an intense conflict that he thought was universal, the 'core complex', consisting of a desire for merger and blissful union with the object, anxiety about being taken over by the object and losing the self and aggression towards the object that arouses such feelings. To withdraw would threaten loss of the object, isolation and depression. Glasser suggests that in those who go on to develop perversions, the solution that is found to this conflict is to sexualise the aggression and to treat the object in a sadistic way, thus maintaining a relationship to the object but finding a means of expressing the intense hostility aroused by the desirable object.

The idea that perverse sexual behaviours may be underpinned by sadomasochism rather than libido is therefore not new; nevertheless the notion that online sexual offending is often underpinned by sadomasochism rather than libido warrants exploration because this notion is so counter to prevailing public attitudes to such phenomena; even with a psychoanalytic framework, it may be important to draw attention to the range of possible unconscious motives for such behaviours and to enquire why the virtual world, and virtual sex in particular, lends itself to being used as a stage on which to enact this battle with a persecutory internal object.

The patients on whom the current chapter is based have sought voluntary outpatient psychotherapy in a state-funded health clinic; they may differ in profile from repeat offenders found in prison populations, who may be more consistently paedophilic, overtly psychopathic or violent. Among patients seeking psychotherapy, some are clearly driven by overtly sadistic or sexual fantasies relating to children, and others are 'polymorphously perverse', presenting with wide-ranging paraphilias. Thus the particular syndrome described here probably represents a small sub-set of Internet offenders, yet a significant sub-set if this challenges the assumption that viewing of child pornography always implies primary paedophilia.

For reasons of confidentiality and because of the sensitivity of this material, I will not provide case material as evidence, but will draw on a number of cases by way of illustration. A typical presentation for patients of this sort would be that they come to therapy after receiving a conviction for possession of illegal images. Where the offence was deemed less serious in legal terms (relatively small numbers of images of clothed children, erotic posing, or sexual contact between children with no penetrative sexual activity), they might have been given a suspended sentence with a probation order and periodic monitoring by the police; for a first offence deemed more serious, they may have incurred a prison sentence.

It is beyond the scope of this paper to explore in detail what the children viewed in the images signify, and why this particular choice of object, though the literature suggests avenues for consideration. Glasser (1988) suggests that the child may carry the projection of an idealised child on whom the person lavishes idealised parental love; implicit in this is a projection of a deprived child-self needing this 'love', and an implicit sadism and triumph towards the parents who have failed the child. Wood (2010) adds to this the envy and hatred that may be felt towards a child perceived to be pure or desirable, compared to a self felt to be damaged or unwanted. The gender of the child may also be significant; for a man viewing child pornography, an image of a boy may represent an idealised self that may also be the object of envy or hatred; a girl may represent aspects of a despised, feminised self, or a displaced maternal object. But rather than exploring these possible identifications here, I want to focus on what paedophilia *per se* comes to mean for the patient, and the way in which he may use the Internet, in part to assume the identity of a paedophile in order to enact a sadomasochistic relationship to his internal objects.

At first glance the relationship to the Internet might appear to be masochistic, in that it is used to inflict psychological suffering on the self. One patient described how looking at pictures of boys whom he believed to be more attractive than him, people who would never have chosen him as a partner, 'was being cruel, in a way, or self-harming, or "miserabling" myself. I'd feel rejected so I'd look at them and it would make me feel better, briefly, and then it would make me feel more miserable, so I'd look at more pictures to make myself feel better … and make myself more miserable'.

Masochism is a complex subject and attempts to locate it at a specific developmental stage, or to separate it out from sadism, may be misguided. Glasser's (1979) model of the core complex assumes that sadism and masochism are but two sides of the same coin, that neither is primary, and that sadomasochism is founded in the response to intense underlying claustro-agoraphobic anxieties in relation to the primary object. If these core complex anxieties and a sadomasochistic solution to them prevails, this will shape the experience of subsequent developmental stages, lending a particularly sadomasochistic quality to anal and genital functioning. In the patients described here, it has become clear in the course of therapy that the ostensibly 'masochistic' pleasure of doing something that would ultimately harm themselves, actually masked pleasure in the suffering inflicted on the other through their own suffering. The underlying dynamic could therefore be thought of as broadly sadomasochistic, ostensibly masochistic, but psychodynamically, sadistic rather than masochistic in emphasis.

Enacting a sadomasochistic relationship to a persecutory internal object

Just as Freud describes in his reference to 'Criminals from a sense of guilt', a patient describes how the feelings of guilt (on this occasion, guilt about looking at legal pornography) precede and drive a defiant act:

> You're looking at legal pornography and thinking 'What would people think if they knew what I was doing?' and of course they would disapprove, and so, that just opens up this *rocket* where you override yourself, and your sense of yourself, and so this may not be legal but you get carried

> away because you are *already* disapproved of. It's not that it would *provoke* disapproval.

This external authority will also be projected onto the therapist in the transference. Two years after he had been sentenced, this man's probation order came to an end. He came to the next session furious with me for a remark I had made in the previous session, feeling that I was only interested in his offence, that I was trying to incriminate him, and implying that it was a serious shortcoming of mine that I was unable to see how much he had endured and could only view him as an offender, in just the way that society scapegoats child sex offenders. At this moment he was determined to draw me away from thinking about what his pursuit of child imagery had meant, and into a relationship in which he – now the harsh authority – was preaching to me about my insensitivity and limitations as a therapist.

I took up his need to create a relationship in his mind in which he felt misunderstood and aggrieved. I linked this to the watershed of the end of his probation order, and that he had felt that probation and the criminal justice system had kept him under malicious scrutiny, and now that it was gone, he felt very anxious and exposed. He started instead to recreate that feeling with me, that I was out to incriminate him and unable to see how he might feel himself to be a victim. He immediately calmed down and confirmed that he could see this. He went on to talk about how he had been working towards this deadline but now it had passed he had no idea what to do with himself. He didn't know what he wanted to do and never had.

The malicious scrutiny is internal, but when externalised there is an external object the patient can hate that bestows a sense of relief – his anxiety is reduced, though subjectively he feels aggrieved and angry. Without the tension and excitement of this battle there is nothing – no sense of identity and direction.

As the therapy progressed, this man was able to see how he provoked and mocked the internal authority, and described looking for a problem in himself that he could amplify. He described the 'internal voice' as a fierce creature in a cage, which he projected onto the computer screen. By acting in a defiant way he 'rattled its cage', yet, he admitted, it turned out to be bigger than he thought it was. In effect, the creature turned round and bit him, as he was arrested and convicted.

Another patient spoke about how he had always been bullied, 'but part of me … I don't know … is like the Jew putting up my hand in front of the Nazis'.

Thus there is a compulsion to provoke the malicious authority, to draw attention to the self and to become locked in battle; without this there is a feeling of emptiness, of nothing. One man described the pleasure of thwarting this internal object by making himself into nothing:

> If I feel someone else is making judgments about me, then I feel I have to submit to that, and it all goes back to the judgments that were made

> about me when I was a child. If someone is treating me in that way I feel I have to destroy myself, and before I do there is a feeling of pleasure. I can't explain it. But I feel I must make myself into nothing.

I commented that if he felt misunderstood by me he was going to make me watch while he destroyed himself, which he confirmed, while acknowledging how difficult this was to talk about.

Thus while looking at pornography on the Internet the individual is in his mind locked in battle with a malicious authority with which he compulsively engages in a sadomasochistic way, baiting the object by looking at ever more extreme material, 'rattling its cage', inviting persecution (and prosecution), but also torturing the object by destroying himself in front of it. The destruction of himself that is enacted here is to make himself into a paedophile, knowing he will be reviled by society. In this way he enacts the unconscious sense of guilt, making himself into a person he imagines will be despised and punished; at the same time, he imagines he is taking control of the situation in which he is subject to persecution, and so derives a perverse feeling of triumph from the destruction of himself.

Filling an intolerable space

What is evident is the almost limitless versatility of this medium to lend itself to enactments of the internal world. Internet sex can serve the vehicle for taking revenge on an object by making the self into something despised and reviled, denied of standing and respect within society. In addition to this, it can serve as a disturbing object that intrudes into the mind to fill an empty space, or the soothing object that obliterates space.

The patient quoted above described making himself into nothing to punish the other who was felt to be misunderstanding or harsh. The provocation of the persecutory object can also be a way of drawing in or engaging an object felt to be unavailable, filling a space felt to be bleak, or giving shape and definition to subjective states felt to be shapeless and empty. Bollas (1996) describes how in borderline personalities, either because they were intrinsically disturbed as infants, or because the early object world was disturbing, in place of a primary object there is an experience of emotional turbulence or disruptive affect. In order to recreate this primary experience the person seeks turbulence, has a 'desire for turbulence', because without this there is the empty space 'following the other's vanishing' (p. 7). He observes, 'The catastrophic feels enlivening' (p. 7). Many of Bollas' observations about such borderline states fit with the use made of the Internet to view illegal pornography. He describes how borderline patients are 'into mind fucking … molesting their own psychic life with overwhelmingly disturbed thoughts' (p.6). This echoes patients' descriptions of their mental state when viewing child pornography: whether or not they are in a state of sexual excitement, they feel highly anxious and disturbed, but the pursuit of this state is compelling because without it there is a profound sense of emptiness or isolation. The turbulence, in effect, fills their minds with sexual and aggressive thoughts. While the images viewed may be of a child being molested, it is also their own psychic life that is being molested and disturbed, as Bollas describes.

In a more passive way, pornography can also be experienced as a 'balm' to foster a kind of mindlessness, which soothes or anaesthetises acute feelings of loneliness, and psychic pain:

> the persecution is gone – and actually there is no thought at all. There's no pain, no suffering, no sadness. And there is no loss. No loss at all. And sometimes when I looked at pictures there was a sexual thing going on and sometimes there wasn't. It could have been legal or illegal. I didn't even notice which. I wasn't thinking at all.

Defiance and surrender to a potentially castrating paternal object

One of these patients described his father as someone who 'seemed to be encouraging and supporting me but as soon as I raised my sail he'd knock it down'. In a further session he described his use of the Internet to enact defiance of this disapproving paternal authority, and the urge to ridicule the paternal authority by imitating but mocking it:

> The offence, was like taking that superego (sic) control and turning it on its head. Like kids going into a sweetshop when they have a very strict Maths teacher – and they take sweets and share them out, two for you, two for me, doing what they would do in a Maths lesson, but actually they are somewhere they shouldn't be, doing something they shouldn't be doing. And it was like that with me. In my head my father's voice is saying 'you can't do this' and 'you can't do that' and there's me doing the same – on the Internet I can look at this and I can't look at that.

I suggested that, because of what he was looking at, he was making a mockery of that voice, with which he agreed.

By making the self into 'nothing' as described previously, and by courting the censure of the law and society, it is possible to see how a man can attack his own potency, knock down his own sail, and, in effect, punish the father by creating a son who can't sail his own boat. Acknowledging that he was driven more by an urge to do something transgressive and defiant than a sexual urge, one patient told me, 'And on the Internet, what can you pick? Paedophilia or terrorism – and now there is extreme pornography, but that wasn't well-publicized at the time'.

The significance of paedophilia in this context is that it is transgressive and abhorrent, the vehicle for the enactment of a sadistic attack on the patient and his objects, rather than principally an expression of desire. The elaboration of sexual fantasies about children can be seen as a very specific attack on an Oedipal father, whose place it is to uphold generational boundaries and the incest taboo. Underlying this attack on the Oedipal father, a fantasised attack on a vulnerable child may represent an attack on an earlier paternal or parental object, experienced as depriving or neglectful.

The patient quoted above, who felt that his sail had been knocked down, also imagined that, like him, I was rendered impotent, in thrall to a powerful man. On one occasion I took up his feeling that either I had no authority, or he experienced me as very directive. He went on to describe a recurrent thought that just before his session I had been with a man in my room who was senior to me, who knew about him, and who told me what line to pursue, and then that is what I did. I pointed out that he put himself and me in the same position of not having that masculine authority for ourselves, and how that left him unable to imagine how he would ever gain that authority through therapy with me. Thus both I and the work of therapy were 'castrated', and no-one could set sail.

The role of the internet in the mind

In 'The economic problem of masochism', Freud (1924) describes how:

> masochism creates a temptation to perform 'sinful' actions which must then be expiated by the reproaches of the sadistic conscience … or by chastisement from the great parental power of Destiny. In order to provoke punishment from this last representative of the parents, the masochist must do what is inexpedient, must act against his own interests, must ruin the prospects which open out to him in the real world and must, perhaps, destroy his own real existence.
>
> (pp. 424–425)

For a proportion of people who have sought out child pornography online, this urge to provoke punishment or chastisement from the sadistic conscience, or its external representatives, the criminal justice system or 'Destiny', can indeed have disastrous consequences, severely curtailing relationship and employment opportunities, impacting on their relationship with children of their own or others, and marking them with the stigma and restrictions of being on the sex offenders' register.

Freud (1916) saw the guilt that might underpin criminal acts as deriving from the Oedipus Complex, 'and was a reaction to the two great criminal intentions of killing the father and having sexual relations with the mother' (p. 333). In contemporary psychoanalytic thought, guilt would be seen as occurring in different forms reflecting different levels of psychic functioning, with persecutory guilt originating in the earlier and more primitive functioning associated with the paranoid-schizoid position, and imbuing the superego with qualities of harshness and ferocity. In the domain of compulsive sexual behaviours and perversions, where full Oedipal functioning has not been achieved, the superego is unlikely to be encountered in the Freudian, 'neurotic' form. Instead, the superego is often more akin to Bion's (1962) 'super-ego' or O'Shaughnessey's (1999) 'abnormal superego' – triumphant, destructive of links, 'an envious assertion of moral superiority without any morals' (Bion, 1962). As the individual develops through the Oedipal stage the paternal object may then assume an extremely persecutory, castrating quality, experienced as both denying the boy a masculine identity, and subjecting him to scorn and humiliation for failing to acquire this. It is this primitive and persecutory object, which in turn dominates oral, anal and phallic phases, which is evident in patients of this type. The defiant act is then not simply an assertion of Oedipal guilt, but a response to primitive guilt with roots in earlier stages of development.

Why, then, should the individuals described here, who ostensibly live under the shadow of a strict and punitive superego and who may never have been arrested or convicted before, enact this urge to transgress on the Internet? The term 'Internet' is used as though this were a static thing, but in the mind it seems to function in three ways: as an object with perceived attributes; as a stage on which internal dramas can be enacted; and as a medium that by virtue of its characteristics, acts as a catalyst, changing the nature of the relationship of the individual to the materials being accessed.

Firstly, as an object with perceived attributes, the distinguishing characteristic of the Internet is its versatility. The Internet creates, par excellence, a screen for projections – not a blank screen as it is so full of content, but a 'screen' so multifaceted and malleable that it lends itself to whatever the individual needs it to be. The Internet may be, simultaneously, experienced as endorsing transgression, seductively inviting corrupt enactments, and embodying a hidden authority waiting to pounce. It may be experienced as mechanical and impersonal, and yet almost humanly communicative and interactive. Like a large group, the virtual community may be seen as a powerful force for good, or as anarchic and dominated by primitive and savage currents. Because it is so multifaceted, there is no one 'reality' to be asserted to counter projections. When interacting with another person, projective mechanisms will sooner or later be challenged by confrontation with the other's reality; on the Internet, such confrontations can be avoided indefinitely. It is clear that we are only just beginning to become aware of the range of disturbed relationships that can be forged in relation to the Internet.

The second role the Internet may have within the mind relates to the Internet's capacity to function as a stage for the enactment of internal dramas, as an extension of its multifaceted, 'polymorphous' nature. It is not merely an object to be projected onto, but invites the individual to participate as an actor, creating whatever drama is desired. Fundamentally, paraphilic behaviours create scenarios in the person's mind, with actors and dramas, and those scenarios function as a means of evacuating intolerable feelings, enacting punishments on the self and others either in fantasy or in reality, avoiding the perils of genuine intimacy with another, and filling unbearable empty spaces in the person's emotional world with excitement. On the Internet the individual can create a virtual 'second life', but also in less concrete ways, the person can engage with sexual scenarios that allow the projection into another of any feelings or parts of the self felt to be intolerable.

The third role that the Internet may come to assume for the psyche is as a catalyst, potentially undermining and even fostering a breakdown in ego functioning in vulnerable individuals. Features of the Internet fuel manic defences, and lead to a breakdown of 'depressive position' functioning (Wood, 2007, 2011). The speed and scale of the Internet, the illusion of control that is fostered, the ability to treat the other as an object with no regard for their subjective experience, the ability to create an idealised image of the self and the illusion that this is not 'real' so no harm is done, all fuel omnipotence, triumph and the denial of limitations, dependency and the potentially harmful effects of one's own aggression. The engagement with a fantasy other can offer an escape from the anxieties of intimacy.

The compulsive use of Internet pornography and online sex is often discussed with no reference to the fact that the sexual act, alongside the evocation of sexual fantasy, usually consists of masturbation. Coen (1981) usefully details the psychic functions of normal masturbation in men: first, it generates feelings of vitality, self-definition and self-cohesion; it provides an illusory presence of another person, restoring a sense of the presence of a comforting mother; it offers omnipotent control; it allows the illusory actualisation of fantasies plus serves as a defence against hostile aggression. There is a striking concordance between these psychic mechanisms engendered by masturbation *per se*, and those processes that seem to render Internet sex particularly compelling. The wealth of material on the Internet, the responsiveness of the Internet and the power this material has to excite, mean that Internet sex can provide a welcome antidote to feelings of emotional deadness or emptiness. The Internet can provide relief from loneliness through a fantasised engagement with an imaginary other, the evocation of an imaginary group or community of which the individual feels themselves to be a part. The individual has access to vast amounts of information at extraordinary speeds, yet can terminate any unwanted exchange at the click of a mouse, fuelling feelings of omnipotent control. Because this is 'virtual' and not 'real', the individual is enabled to feel that harmful, aggressive feelings enacted through sexual fantasies are rendered innocuous. Thus the particular attributes of the Internet amplify those functions of masturbation documented by Coen, to generate a powerful and seductive mix. Like masturbation, Internet sex only offers a temporary solution to these conflicts, hence the potential for a repetitive, addictive relationship.

It also seems crucially important that engagement with the Internet can be experienced as being on the border between internal and external reality, both more different and hence more exciting than simply an elaboration of unconscious fantasy, but also accessed in privacy, with no witnesses, and under the individual's control, in a way that can be experienced as though it is simply an extension of the individual's own mind. Bollas (1996) notes that borderline patients seek 'borderline objects', objects that enable them 'to conjure self-afflicting turbulence at any time', and so exist on the border of the external and the internal, 'linked to an external happening, yet immediately evocative internally' (p.7). The Internet, or Internet sex, through the medium of disturbing sexual imagery, can function as just such a borderline object, which can be relied on to evoke the turbulence of sexual excitement, guilt about sexual, aggressive and transgressive impulses and fear of retribution, but all under the individual's control.

This position on the border of external and internal reality may also have a vital significance with respect to ego and superego controls. It could be argued that the dynamics described here could equally be enacted with an actual child, rather than Internet images of a child, and that there is nothing unique about the contribution of accessing sexual materials on the Internet; an actual child could be used to enact transgression and sadomasochism, to externalise an internal drama, and as a screen or a vessel for projections and projective identification. But to commit a sexual assault on an actual child would require far greater overriding of observed reality, and the violent breaching of another's body. The patients described here have no history of violence and are inhibited rather than disinhibited in the expression of aggression. They would be very unlikely to commit a violent sexual assault against a child, or even, pre-Internet, to have actively sought out child pornography.

In all of us the ego and superego seem to have one set of rules regulating things designated 'fantasy' in the mind, which might permit thoughts of perverse, violent or inhumane acts, and another set of rules governing actions. Much more lenient rules usually operate where fantasies are concerned. For some individuals, the use of the Internet, seeming to be on the boundary of the internal and the external, appears to call into play the implicit rules relating to 'fantasy' rather than those governing 'actions'. Thus individuals may be shocked when arrested, believing themselves only to have enacted something in their minds. One patient was indignant that he had been convicted of a 'thought crime' as in Orwell's novel *1984* (1949).

The Internet may also come to be equated with a corrupt authority in the person's mind. Some websites are structured in such a way as to draw the individual in to view ever more extreme materials. The Internet, or clusters of people in forums or chatrooms, may also come to symbolise an invisible group.

Freud's (1921) account of people's behaviour in unstructured, ephemeral groups is strikingly similar to the behaviour reported by some people using Internet sex. Freud describes how:

> when individuals come together in a group, all of their individual inhibitions fall away and all the cruel, brutal and destructive instincts, which lie dormant in individuals as relics of a primitive epoch, are stirred up to find free gratification.
>
> (1921, p. 79)

The Internet creates the illusion of a group of people who share the same sexual interests, but these are unstructured, ephemeral groups as Freud describes: in chatrooms there may be a recognisable 'group' of participants, but more commonly on the Internet the boundaries of the group are undefined, the membership is fluid and behavioural codes are vague. The individual's normal ego and superego controls may be relinquished or subordinated to an investment in this imagined group, which seems to promise endless sexual gratification without constraint or judgment. While many web-based communities have high ideals and function more like the 'structured' groups Freud refers to, which can generate the highest human achievements, people engaging with online sex can easily be drawn to virtual groups that endorse transgression, regression to pre-genital forms of sexuality and the fantasised enactment of destructiveness.

Concluding remarks

What are the implications of viewing the use of child pornography as, in part, an enactment of a sadomasochistic or 'borderline' internal object in the way that has been described? It is clear that the patients I have described experienced this act of transgression as an exciting, defiant enactment and provocation, filling a terrifying internal space. They also experienced their own illegal behaviour as a cry for help, a signal of the danger they felt themselves to be in. At the conscious and preconscious level, what they were aware of was a sense of danger associated with the persecutory internal object, their extreme self-criticism and self disgust, or the projection of this onto society. However, underlying this sense of danger from persecution there is the more profound, and more unconscious fear of the engulfing emptiness of a primary object, which failed to protect or satisfy. At one time they are both identified with the sadistic condemnation of themselves, and the victim of that condemnation; they are in danger from an appalling sense of emptiness and isolation, and the agent who can magically fill that space with 'tumult' (in Bollas' terms) and sexual excitement. Patients describe a spiralling lack of control. Perhaps it is this sense of danger that leads them to behave recklessly if not provocatively, in some cases inviting detection.

The downloading of child pornography, like any other symptom, will be overdetermined. The specific images sought will have significance for the individual, and will probably have multiple meanings. Only one facet of such behaviour has been considered here, but it is an aspect that is salient in some individuals seeking psychotherapy: the deliberate use of illegal images on the Internet to enact transgression and defiance. In this situation, breaking the law, breaching social codes and inviting vilification is not incidental to, or the price to be paid for the enactment of desire, but is a principal and motivating force in the behaviour. The Internet does not only lend itself for use as a medium in this enactment; its very characteristics may be felt by some individuals to invite such enactments.

References

Bion, W.R. (1962) *Learning from experience*. London: Karnac.

Bollas, C. (1996) Borderline desire. *International Forum of Psychoanalysis*, *5*(1), 5–9.

Coen, S.J. (1981) Sexualization as a predominant mode of defense. *Journal of the American Psychoanalytic Association*, *29*, 893–921.

Freud, S. (1905) Three essays on the theory of sexuality. *Standard Edition*, *7*, 125–243.

Freud, S. (1916) Some character types met with in psychoanalytic work. *Standard Edition*, *14*, 311–333.

Freud, S. (1919) A child is being beaten. *Standard Edition*, *17*, 177–243.

Freud, S. (1921) Group psychology and the analysis of the ego. *Standard Edition, 18*, 65–143.

Freud, S. (1924) The economic problem of masochism. *Standard Edition*, *19*, 155–170.

Freud, S. (1927) Fetishism. *Standard Edition, 21*, 149–157.

Gillespie, W.H. (1940) A contribution to the study of fetishism. *International Journal of Psycho-Analysis, 21*, 401–415.

Gillespie, W.H. (1956) The structure and aetiology of sexual perversion. In S. Lorand and M. Balint (Eds) *Perversions: Psychodynamics in therapy*. New York: Random House. Reproduced in M.D.A. Sinason (Ed.) (1995) *Life, sex and death: Selected writings of W.H. Gillespie*. New Library of Psychoanalysis. London: Routledge.

Glasser, M. (1979) Some aspects of the role of aggression in the perversions. In I. Rosen (Ed.) *Sexual deviation* (2nd edition). Oxford: OUP.

Glasser, M. (1988) Psychodynamic aspects of paedophilia. *Psychoanalytic Psychotherapy*, *3*(2), 121–135.

Glover, E. (1933) The relation of perversion formation to the development of the reality sense. *International Journal of Psycho-Analysis*, *14*, 486–504.

Middleton, D., Mandeville-Norton, R., and Hayes, E. (2009) Does treatment work with internet sex offenders? Emerging findings from the Internet Sex offender treatment programme (i-SOTP). *Journal of Sexual Aggression, 15*, 5–9.

Orwell, G. (1949) *1984*. London: Martin Secker and Warburg Ltd. Reprinted Penguin Books, 1954.

O'Shaughnessey, E. (1999) Relating to the superego. *International Journal of Psychoanalysis*, *80*, 861–870.

Payne, S. (1939) Some observations on the ego development of the fetishist. *International Journal of Psychoanalysis, 20*, 161–170.

Stoller, R. (1975) *Perversion: The erotic form of hatred.* London: Quartet.
Taylor, M. and Quayle, E. (2003) *Child pornography: An internet crime.* Hove: Bruner Routledge.
Wood, H. (2007) Compulsive use of internet pornography: Addiction or perversion? In D. Morgan and S. Ruszczynski (Eds) *Lectures on violence, perversion and delinquency.* London: Karnac.
Wood, H. (2010) Applied psychoanalytic work in forensic settings: The understanding and treatment of paedophilia. In A. Lemma and M. Patrick (Eds) *Off the couch: Contemporary psychoanalytic applications.* London: Routledge.
Wood, H. (2011) The role of the internet in the escalation of sexually compulsive behaviour. *Psychoanalytic Psychotherapy, 25*(2), 127–142.

Index